Top 100 Drugs: CPhT Edition for PTCE and ExCPT

❖ First Edition, 2025
❖ Copyright 2025, CaferMed LLC
❖ Author: Jason Cafer MD
❖ ISBN: 978-1-7350901-7-7
❖ Contact: jason@cafermed.com

Medication Mascots

❖ Mnemonic engineering
➤ Each drug is represented by a distinctive character designed to encode key information
❖ Name-based visual mnemonics
➤ Most mascots are derived from a phrase linking the generic and brand name
◇ Atorvastatin (LIPITOR) → "Lippy Tornado"
◇ Metformin (GLUCOPHAGE) → "Mr. Met formin' Glucose Fudge"
❖ Purpose: Cognitive anchoring
➤ Provides mental hooks for remembering pharmacologic concepts
➤ Uses visual memory to support fast, durable recall in real-world settings
❖ Advanced applications
➤ In higher-level CaferMed books, mascots evolve into data-driven interaction avatars
◇ Designed to help prescribers and pharmacists visualize specific drug-drug interactions

Medications Included

❖ This book was written in 2025 using the most recent Top 300 Drugs list from clincalc.com
➤ The data is based on the Medical Expenditure Panel Survey (MEPS) prescribed medicines file for the year 2022
❖ Additional medication mascots are available at cafermed.com/subscribe

About the Author

❖ Dr. Jason Cafer (pronounced KAY-fur) is an Assistant Professor of Clinical Psychiatry at the University of Missouri–Columbia.
❖ He serves as the inpatient supervising psychiatrist at the Missouri Psychiatric Center.
❖ He is the author of Cafer's Psychopharmacology: Visualize to Memorize 300 Medication Mascots, a book designed for prescribers and pharmacists, yet accessible to students.

Definitions & High-Yield Topics

Anticholinergic Side Effects

❖ Caused by drugs that block acetylcholine, a key body chemical (neurotransmitter)

❖ Named "anticholinergic" because they oppose (anti-) cholinergic (acetylcholine) activity

❖ Acetylcholine controls things like digestion, urination, vision, and sweating

❖ Blocking it leads to side effects described by the classic mnemonic:

  ➤ "Hot as a hare" – Fever, reduced sweating

  ➤ "Dry as a bone" – Dry mouth and skin

  ➤ "Red as a beet" – Flushed skin

  ➤ "Blind as a bat" – Blurred vision, dilated pupils

  ➤ "Mad as a hatter" – Confusion, delirium

❖ Older adults are more sensitive to anticholinergic side effects

❖ Anticholinergic medications among the Top 100:

  ➤ Amitriptyline (#87) > Hydroxyzine (#46) > Paroxetine (#92)

❖ Alternate mnemonics:

  ➤ "Can't see, can't pee, can't spit, can't…poop."

  ➤ "Everything dry"

  ➤ "Tacky Auntie Choli" – "tacky" refers to tachycardia (fast heart rate)

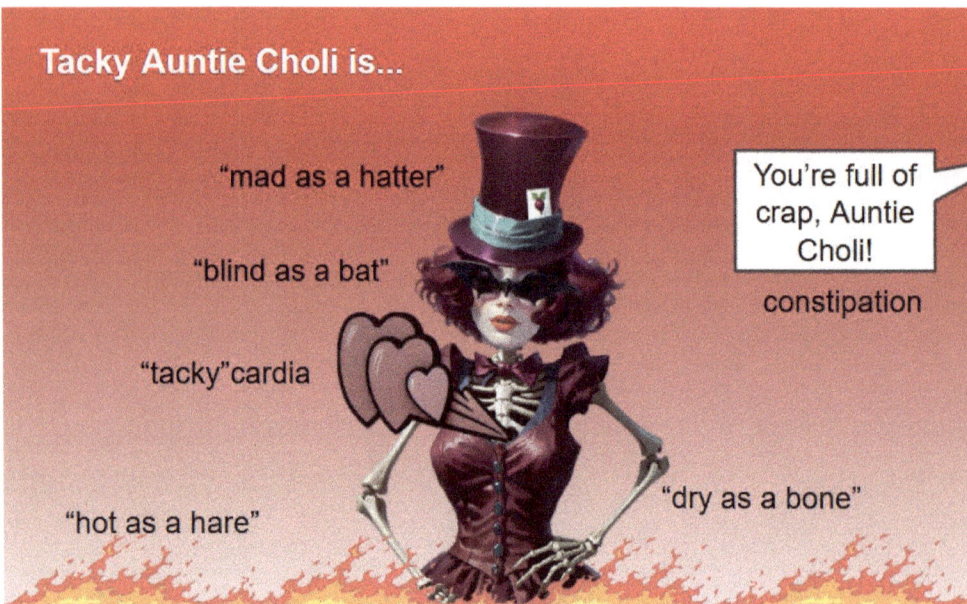

Tacky Auntie Choli is...

"mad as a hatter"

"blind as a bat"

"tacky"cardia

"hot as a hare"

You're full of crap, Auntie Choli!

constipation

"dry as a bone"

Benzodiazepine Withdrawal

❖ Happens when stopping benzodiazepines (benzos) after regular or long-term use

❖ Can be dangerous — unlike opioid or serotonin withdrawal, which are uncomfortable but not life-threatening

❖ Nearly identical to alcohol withdrawal

➤ Benzos and alcohol both act on GABA-A receptors in the brain

❖ Symptoms: anxiety, insomnia, tremors, sweating, irritability, muscle pain

❖ In severe cases: seizures or hallucinations

➤ Called "delirium tremens" when due to alcohol; the term isn't used for benzos, but the physiology is the same

❖ It is safer to taper benzos very slowly, often over weeks to months

❖ Higher risk with high doses or short-acting benzos like Alprazolam (Xanax)

❖ Benzos in the Top 100:

➤ Alprazolam (#41), Clonazepam (#57), and Lorazepam (#81)

➤ Zolpidem (#66) is benzo-like, with lower dependence risk due to nighttime use only

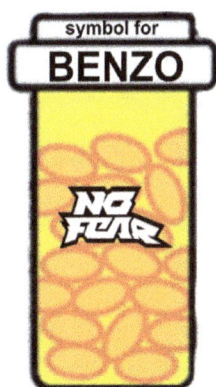

symbol for BENZO
NO FEAR

Alprazolam (XANAX)

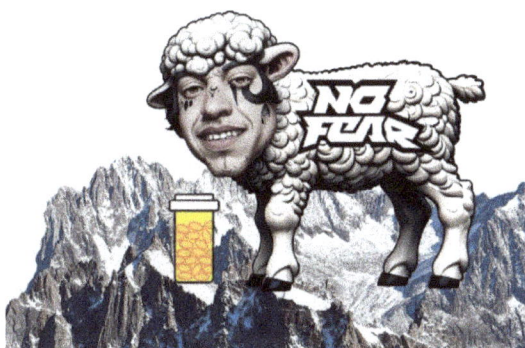

Clonazepam (KLONOPIN)

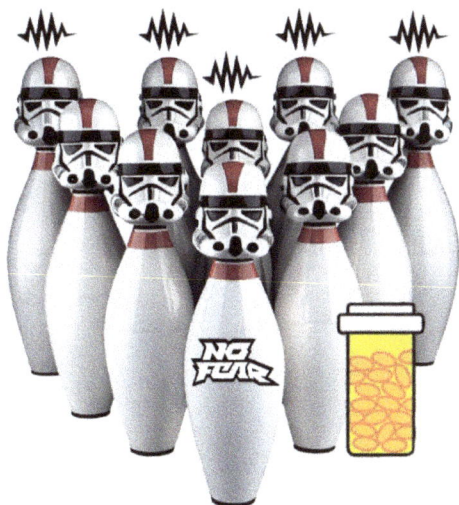

Ativan (LORAZEPAM)

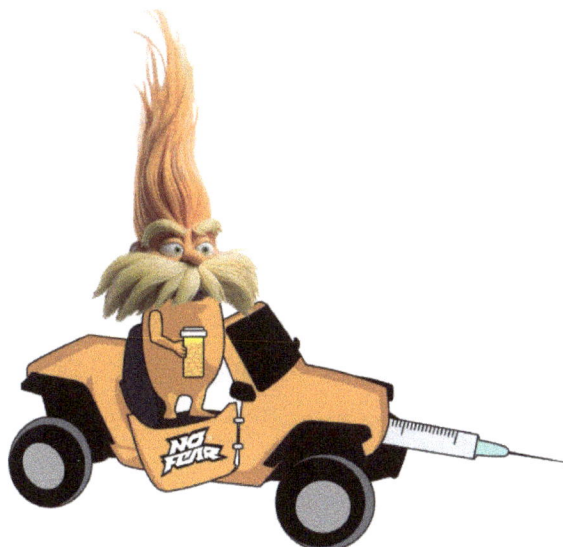

Boxed Warning

❖ Also called a "black box warning"

❖ Strongest warning the Food & Drug Administration (FDA) requires on a medication label

❖ Highlights life-threatening risks

❖ Appears at the top of the drug's prescribing info, inside a bold box

❖ Boxed warnings among Top 100 drugs, ranked roughly by clinical significance and relevance in real-world practice (although all are important):

Boxed Warning	Medications	Details
Bleeding risk	Warfarin (#85) Apixaban (#27) Rivaroxaban (#90) Clopidogrel (#47)	Including intracranial and GI bleeding; Requires INR monitoring (warfarin) or renal dosing (apixaban, rivaroxaban)
Opioid addiction, abuse, and respiratory depression; Risk of fatal overdose is especially high when combined with benzodiazepines or alcohol	Oxycodone (#60, #98) Hydrocodone (#23) Tramadol (#55)	Very high risk for oxycodone and hydrocodone (Schedule II controlled substance); Much lower risk for tramadol (Schedule IV)
Stevens-Johnson Syndrome (SJS) – life-threatening illness starting with a rash; Called toxic epidermal necrolysis (TEN) if severe rash covers >30% of body surface	Lamotrigine (#58)	Patients should contact their prescriber immediately if any rash develops; Lamotrigine should be discontinued at the first sign of rash (unless the rash is clearly not drug related)
Risks include abuse, addiction, withdrawal, and fatal interaction with opioids	Alprazolam (#41) Clonazepam (#57) Lorazepam (#81)	Benzos increase risk of fatal opioid overdose 4- to 10-fold; 31% of opioid overdose deaths involved a benzo (FDA, 2017)
Risk of fetal injury when ACE inhibitors or Angiotensin II receptor blockers (ARBs) are used in pregnancy during second or third trimester	Lisinopril (#3, #53) Losartan (#8) Olmesartan (#97)	Applies to all medications that directly inhibit the renin-angiotensin system (RAAS); Stop as soon as pregnancy is detected
Estrogens increase the risk of	Estradiol (#50)	Unopposed estrogen (i.e.,

endometrial cancer and may raise the risk of stroke, myocardial infarction, venous thromboembolism, and dementia, especially in postmenopausal women	-Not paired with a progestin Ethinyl Estradiol (#80, #99) -Paired with a progestin	estrogen given without a progestin) increases the risk of endometrial cancer in women of any age who have a uterus
Risk of thyroid C-cell tumors	Semaglutide (#48) Dulaglutide (#74)	GLP-1 agonist class warning; Based on rodent studies – relevance to humans is unclear
Increased mortality in elderly patients with dementia-related psychosis	Quetiapine (#82)	Applies to all antipsychotics
Risk of abuse, dependence, and serious cardiovascular events with stimulants	Adderall (#14) Methylphenidate (#32) Lisdexamfetamine (#69)	Schedule II controlled substances; In real-world practice abuse and diversion (selling or sharing stimulants with others) is more common than addiction or heart problems
Suicidal thoughts and behaviors in children, adolescents, and young adults < age 25	Sertraline (#11) Escitalopram (#15) Fluoxetine (#22) Citalopram (#40) Paroxetine (#92) Duloxetine (#31) Venlafaxine (#44) Bupropion (#21) Amitriptyline (#87) Quetiapine (#82)	Applies to all medications approved for the treatment of major depressive disorder (MDD), not just drugs classified as "antidepressants"; The boxed warning is required even if no increased suicidality was observed for the specific drug in trials
Asthma-related deaths associated with long-acting beta 2 agonist (LABA) inhalers	Salmeterol (#59) – Paired with ICS fluticasone Formoterol (#83) – Paired with ICS budesonide There are no LABA monotherapy (single drug) inhalers (e.g., salmeterol or formoterol alone) in the Top 300 drugs	The risk is linked to LABA monotherapy, and does not apply when a LABA is combined with an inhaled corticosteroid (ICS). Still, the FDA mandates a boxed warning on all LABA-containing products due to this class effect, even if combined with ICS.

CNS Depression

❖ Stands for Central Nervous System depressant
❖ Slows brain activity → causes drowsiness, slowed breathing, reduced alertness
❖ Includes benzodiazepines, opioids, alcohol, sleep meds, and some muscle relaxants
❖ Combining CNS depressants can be dangerous — risk of overdose, coma, or death

Contraindication

❖ A specific situation or condition in which a treatment should not be used because it may be harmful to the patient
❖ ABSOLUTE contraindications – must not be used under any circumstance:
  ➤ ACE inhibitors in pregnancy – risk of fetal injury or death
    ◇ Lisinopril (#3)
  ➤ GLP-1 receptor agonists in patients with medullary thyroid carcinoma or Multiple Endocrine Neoplasia type 2 (MEN2)
    ◇ Semaglutide (#48), Dulaglutide (#74)
  ➤ Metformin in severe renal impairment – risk of lactic acidosis
  ➤ Beta blockers in severe bradycardia (slow heart rate) or heart block (delayed heart conduction)
    ◇ Metoprolol (#6), Carvedilol (#34), Atenolol (#63), Propranolol (#77)
  ➤ Nonsteroidal anti-inflammatory drugs (NSAIDs) in active GI bleeding or peptic ulcer (a sore in stomach lining)
    ◇ Ibuprofen (#33), Naproxen (#89), Meloxicam (#29)
  ➤ Statins in active liver disease or pregnancy
    ◇ Rosuvastatin (#13), Simvastatin (#19), Pravastatin (#37), Lovastatin (#111)
❖ RELATIVE contraindications – should not be used under most circumstances, but may be justified (typically by judgment of a specialist) if the benefits clearly outweigh the risks
  ➤ Bupropion (#21) in seizure disorders and eating disorders – ↑ seizure risk
  ➤ Beta blockers in asthma — possible bronchospasm
    ◇ Lower risk: Metoprolol (#6), Atenolol (#63)
    ◇ Higher risk: Carvedilol (#34), Propranolol (#77)

Controlled Substances

❖ Determined by the Drug Enforcement Administration (DEA)

Schedule	Abuse Potential	Examples	Refills Allowed
C-I	Highest	Heroin, LSD, Ecstasy, Marijuana (Federally)	N/A (illegal substances)
C-II	High	Oxycodone, Morphine, Adderall, Methylphenidate	No refills allowed
C-III	Moderate to high	Tylenol #3, Buprenorphine	Up to 5 refills in 6 months
C-IV	Lower than C-III	Benzodiazepines, Zolpidem, Tramadol	Up to 5 refills in 6 months
C-V	Lowest	Cough syrups with codeine (low dose), Pregabalin	Up to 5 refills in 6 months
Non-controlled	None	NSAIDs, antidepressants, antibiotics, diabetes medications	No limit

"Easily Replaceable?"

❖ Tells you how unique or replaceable a medication is.
❖ If insurance doesn't cover it, can the doctor pick a good alternative?
❖ Substitutions are made by the prescriber, not usually the pharmacist
❖ Automatic pharmacy substitutions are rare in retail, but some hospitals have them (e.g., switching omeprazole to pantoprazole)

Half-life

❖ Time it takes for half the drug to leave the body
❖ Helps determine dosing schedule and how long effects last
❖ Short half-life = leaves body quickly
  ➤ May need more frequent dosing
  ➤ When the medication is stopped, withdrawal symptoms may appear sooner
❖ Long half-life = stays in body longer
  ➤ May need less frequent dosing

Off-Label

❖ When a medication is prescribed for a use not approved by the FDA

❖ It's legal and common — based on clinical judgment

❖ Not bad or unsafe by itself — but use should be based on research and medical guidelines

❖ Some uses are off-label because the drug company didn't apply for FDA approval — approval requires time and money, even if evidence supports the use

❖ Example: Trazodone (#18) is approved for depression but commonly used off-label for insomnia

Opioid Withdrawal

❖ Happens when stopping opioids suddenly after regular use

❖ Not life-threatening, but extremely uncomfortable

❖ Common symptoms: body aches, sweating, chills, nausea, diarrhea, anxiety, runny nose

❖ Often described as "bad flu with extra pain"

❖ Opioids in the Top 100: Hydrocodone (#23), Oxycodone (#60, #98), and Tramadol (#55)

QT Prolongation

❖ A delay in heart's electrical reset between beats (longer QT interval on electrocardiogram)

❖ Can lead to a dangerous rhythm called *torsades de pointes*

❖ Risk increases with certain meds, low potassium or magnesium, or drug interactions

❖ QT prolongation alone rarely causes problems — it's cumulative risk that matters

❖ Among the Top 100 drugs, these prolong QT interval:

➤ Citalopram (#40), Ondansetron (#61), Azithromycin (#78), and Quetiapine (#82)

➤ Even if a patient were taking several of these QT-prolonging meds, the risk of torsades is still low unless they have other risk factors (like low potassium, heart disease, high doses, or other interacting meds)

➤ Some less common meds (>#100) prolong QT more and are higher-risk, such as sotalol and methadone

❖ Most patients won't be affected—don't worry unless multiple high-risk factors or flagged by pharmacist

❖ Mnemonic: "Cutie prolongation"

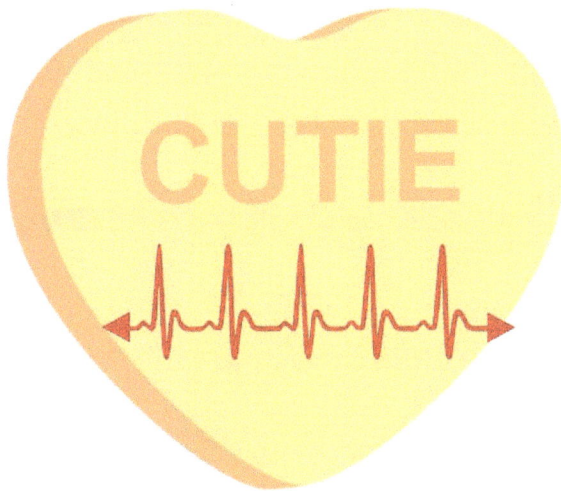

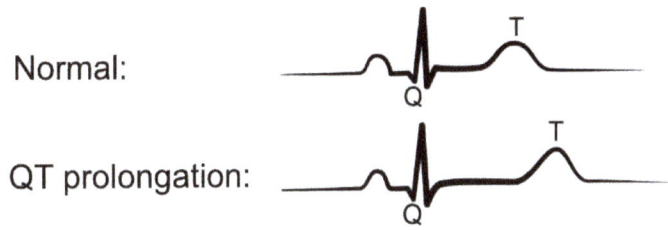

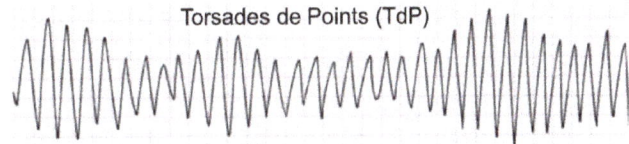

Normal:

QT prolongation:

Torsades de Points (TdP)

Renal Dosing

❖ Renal dosing means adjusting a drug's dose based on the patient's kidney function, typically measured by estimated glomerular filtration rate (eGFR) or creatinine clearance (CrCl)

❖ For drugs eliminated renally (by the kidneys), impaired renal function can lead to drug accumulation and toxicity

❖ Renal dose adjustments may involve lowering the dose or avoiding the drug altogether in severe kidney disease

❖ Top 100 drugs with recommended renal dosing:

➤ Diabetes medications: Metformin (#2), Sitagliptin (#86), Glipizide (#42), Glimepiride (#64), Semaglutide (#48), Dulaglutide (#74), Insulin Glargine (#28), Insulin Aspart (#76), Insulin Lispro (#70)

➤ Anticoagulants / Antiplatelets: Warfarin (#85), Apixaban (#27), Rivaroxaban (#90), Clopidogrel (#47)

➤ Anticonvulsants: Gabapentin (#10), Pregabalin (#91), Lamotrigine (#58), Topiramate (#84)

➤ Cardiovascular meds: Lisinopril (#3), Atenolol (#63), Spironolactone (#52)

➤ SNRI antidepressants: Duloxetine (#31), Venlafaxine (#44)

➤ GI meds: Ondansetron (#61), Famotidine (#49)

➤ Antibiotic: Amoxicillin + Clavulanate (#96)

➤ Lipid-Lowering med: Fenofibrate (#88)

➤ Gout medication: Allopurinol (#39)

➤ Opioid: Oxycodone (#60)

Serotonin Syndrome

❖ More accurately called serotonin toxicity — a rare, often misunderstood effect of overstimulation of serotonin receptors

❖ Symptoms like tremor, sweating, or agitation typically appear within 24 hours of starting or increasing a serotonergic drug

❖ Not caused by long-term use of multiple serotonergic medications

❖ Becomes dangerous when a serotonin reuptake inhibitor (SSRI or SNRI) is combined with a monoamine oxidase inhibitor (MAOI)

❖ Examples of MAOIs: phenelzine, tranylcypromine, isocarboxazid, selegiline, linezolid, methylene blue

❖ MAOIs are rare, so most serotonergic combinations cause only mild side effects, not life-threatening toxicity

❖ The same medications that can cause serotonin toxicity when combined with an MAOI may also cause serotonin withdrawal if stopped abruptly

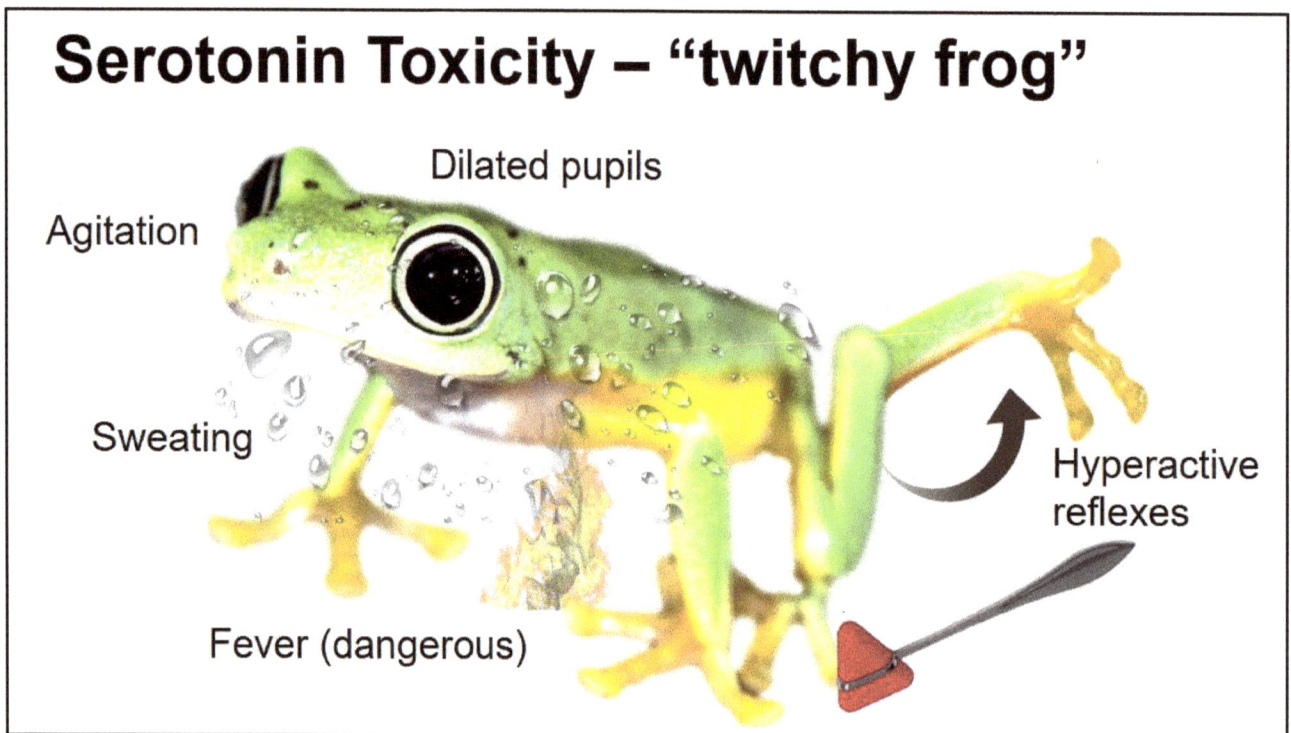

Serotonin Toxicity – "twitchy frog"

Dilated pupils

Agitation

Sweating

Hyperactive reflexes

Fever (dangerous)

Serotonin Withdrawal (Antidepressant Discontinuation Symptoms)

❖ Happens when stopping a serotonin reuptake inhibitor too quickly, applicable to:

➤ Selective serotonin reuptake inhibitors (SSRIs)

➤ Norepinephrine reuptake inhibitors (SNRIs)

❖ Not dangerous, but uncomfortable

❖ Main symptoms: Lightheadedness, paresthesias (tingling sensations), nausea, fatigue, and irritability

❖ May also cause "brain zaps" (electric shock-like feeling) in addition to symptoms described below

❖ More common with short-acting drugs:

➤ Venlafaxine (Effexor) – serotonin and norepinephrine reuptake inhibitor (SNRI)

➤ Paroxetine (Paxil) – selective serotonin reuptake inhibitor (SSRI)

❖ Tapering slowly helps prevent it

❖ Serotonin reuptake inhibitors (SRIs) in the Top 100, strongly associated with serotonin withdrawal:

➤ SSRIs: Sertraline (#11), Escitalopram (#15), Fluoxetine (#22), Citalopram (#40), and Paroxetine (#92)

➤ SNRIs: Duloxetine (#31) and Venlafaxine (#44)

❖ Top 100 medications with SRI properties, less strongly associated with serotonin withdrawal

➤ Tricyclic antidepressant (TCA): Amitriptyline (#87)

➤ Serotonin modulator / atypical antidepressant: Trazodone (#18)

➤ Weak opioid + SNRI: Tramadol (#55)

❖ Top 100 antidepressant without SRI properties – does NOT cause serotonin withdrawal:

➤ Bupropion (#21) – mechanism involves norepinephrine and dopamine, not serotonin

❖ Top 100 medications with serotonin-related mechanisms that do NOT cause serotonin withdrawal because they are not SRIs:

➤ Buspirone (#54), Ondansetron (#61), Quetiapine (#82), and Sumatriptan (#95)

❖ The same medications that can cause serotonin withdrawal may also contribute to serotonin toxicity

Serotonin Discontinuation Symptoms = Antidepressant Withdrawal

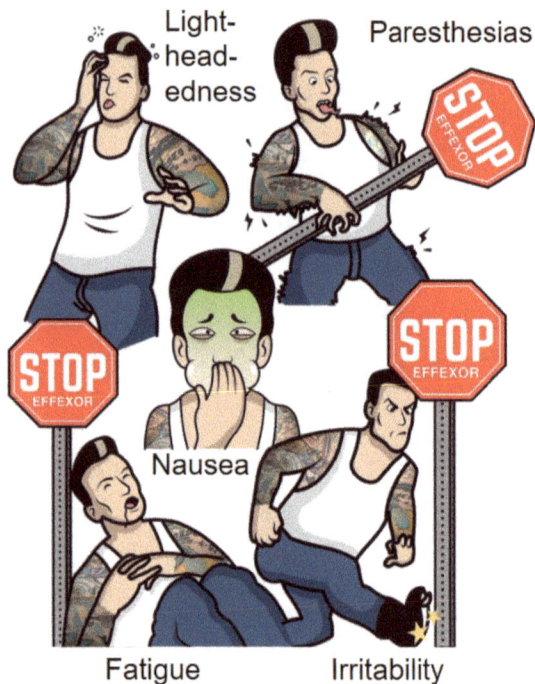

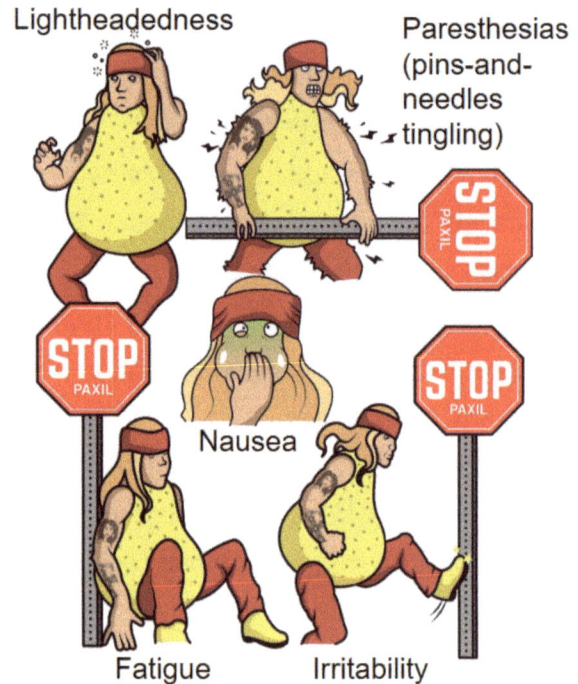

Therapeutic Index (TI)

❖ Safety margin
❖ Ratio between a drug's toxic dose and effective dose
❖ Narrow TI = Risky
  ➤ Toxic dose is not far from effective dose
  ➤ Small difference means dosing must be exact
  ➤ Digoxin, Warfarin, Insulin, Lithium, Cyclosporine, Phenytoin, Potassium, Tacrolimus, Amitriptyline
❖ Wide TI = Safer
  ➤ Toxic dose is much larger than effective dose
  ➤ Big difference allows more flexibility in dosing
  ➤ Penicillin, Cephalexin, Famotidine, Loratadine, Sertraline, Escitalopram, Buspirone, Mirtazapine

#1 Atorvastatin (LIPITOR)

uh-TOR-vuh-stat-in (LIP-ih-tor)
Common Uses: High cholesterol
Mascot: "Lippy Tornado"

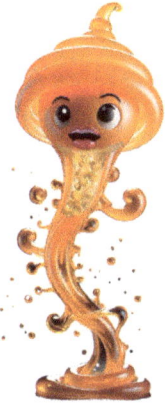

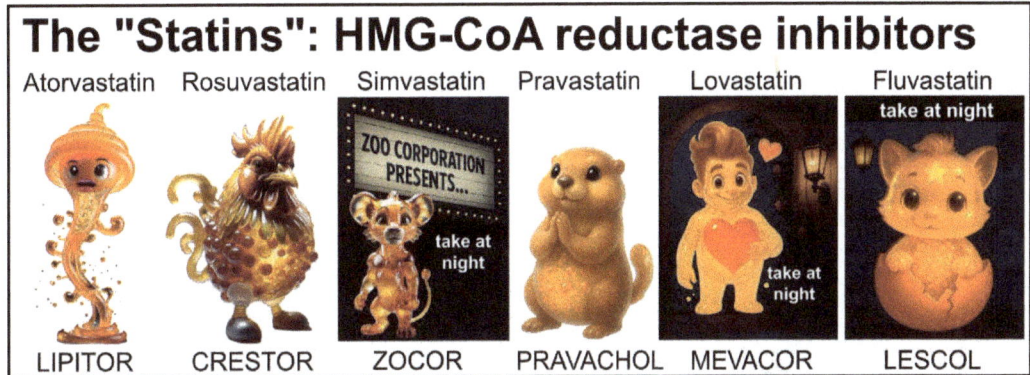

The "Statins": HMG-CoA reductase inhibitors
Atorvastatin — LIPITOR
Rosuvastatin — CRESTOR
Simvastatin (take at night) — ZOCOR
Pravastatin — PRAVACHOL
Lovastatin (take at night) — MEVACOR
Fluvastatin (take at night) — LESCOL

Alternate Mnemonics:

❖ "A-TORpedo to sink LDL (bad) cholesterol"

❖ "Stat-in for fat-in your arteries"

❖ "A tall statin knocks cholesterol down"

❖ "ATOR – A Top Of Range statin" – high potency at 40–80 mg

❖ "ATorvastatin attacks ATherosclerosis"

❖ *Atorvastatin* song available on YouTube, Spotify, etc

Drug Class: Cholesterol-lowering: Statin (HMG-CoA reductase inhibitor)
Similar Statins: Rosuvastatin (#13), Simvastatin (#19), Pravastatin (#37), Lovastatin (#111)
Comparisons: More powerful than simvastatin
High-Alert Risk: ✅ Not high alert
Major Side Effects: Muscle pain, liver problems, rare rhabdomyolysis (muscle breakdown)
Narrow Therapeutic Index: No
Precautions: Avoid with liver problems or grapefruit juice (which increases drug levels)
Routes: Oral
Easily Replaceable? Yes – several other statins are available
Also: Does not need to be taken at bedtime (unlike simvastatin)

Sample Test Questions:
Q: What serious muscle-related condition is a rare side effect of atorvastatin?
A: Rhabdomyolysis – applicable to all statins
Q: Why should grapefruit be avoided while taking atorvastatin?
A: Grapefruit increases atorvastatin levels

#2 Metformin (GLUCOPHAGE)

MET-for-min (GLOO-koh-fahj)

Common Uses: Type 2 diabetes, weight management

Mascot: "Mr Met formin' Glucose Fudge"

➤ The fudge is shaped like mitochondria, where metformin acts

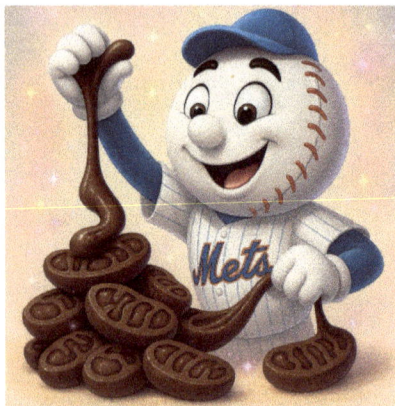

Alternate Mnemonics:

❖ "Met forms glucose tolerance" – improves glucose sensitivity of cells

❖ "Glucophage gulps the glucose" – phage means "eat"

❖ *Metformin* song available on YouTube, Spotify, etc

➤ *Metformin, Glucophage, big ol' Biguanide, won't make you bigger, weight may decline*

Drug Class: Diabetes medication: Biguanide – Metformin is the only available biguanide

Similar Drugs: None (except nutritional supplement berberine)

Comparisons: First choice for type 2 diabetes; causes less weight loss than GLP-1 agonists

High-Alert Risk: ⚠ Risk of lactic acidosis if kidney problems, dehydration, or large overdose

Major Side Effects: Stomach upset, diarrhea, vitamin B12 deficiency

➤ Does not cause hypoglycemia (low blood sugar) like some diabetes medications

Look-Alike/Sound-Alike: Metronidazole

Narrow Therapeutic Index: No

Precautions: Avoid in poor kidney function; stop before contrast scans

Routes: Oral

Easily Replaceable? No – no other medications work the same way

Also: ER (extended-release) forms cause less stomach upset and diarrhea

Sample Test Questions:

Q: What rare side effect can occur in people with poor kidney function?

A: Lactic acidosis

Q: Should metformin be stopped before a CT scan with contrast?

A: Yes

#3 Lisinopril (Zestril)

lih-SIN-oh-pril (ZESS-tril)
Common Uses: Hypertension (high blood pressure), heart failure, after heart attack
Mascot: "Licensed Zest drill"

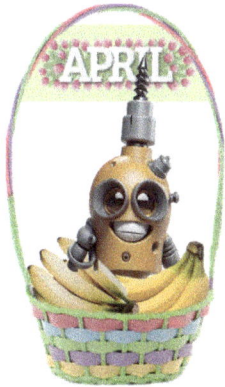

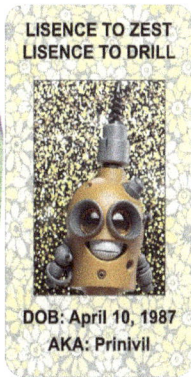

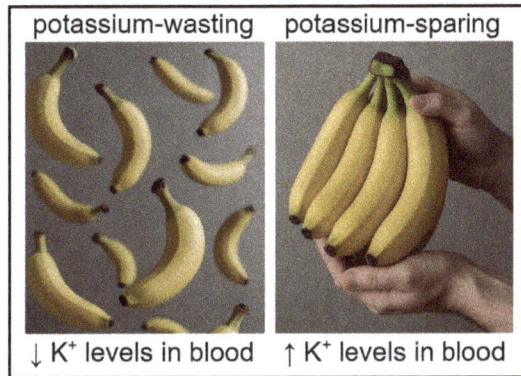

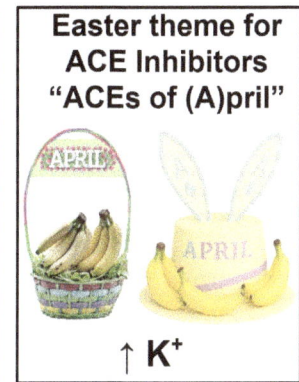

LISENCE TO ZEST
LISENCE TO DRILL

DOB: April 10, 1987
AKA: Prinivil

potassium-wasting ↓ K$^+$ levels in blood

potassium-sparing ↑ K$^+$ levels in blood

Easter theme for ACE Inhibitors "ACEs of (A)pril"

↑ K$^+$

Alternate mnemonics:

❖ "Listen—your blood pressure just dropped!"

❖ "-prils put pressure in its place"

❖ "ACE up the sleeve against hypertension"

❖ "Lisino-chill pill for the arteries"

❖ "PRIL = Pressure Regulating Inhibitor of Lungs" – cough is a side effect of ACE inhibitors

❖ *ACE Inhibitors* song available on YouTube, Spotify, etc

Drug Class: Blood pressure medication: Angiotensin Converting Enzyme (ACE) inhibitor
Similar Drugs: Enalapril (#141), Ramipril (#187), Lisinopril/Hydrocholothiazide combo (#53)
Comparisons: Similar to angiotensin II receptor blockers (ARBs, -sartans)

➤ ARBs are often used instead if cough with ACE inhibitors is a problem

High-Alert Risk: ✅ Not high alert
Major Side Effects: Dry cough, high potassium, swelling of lips or throat
Look-Alike/Sound-Alike: Lisdexamfetamine (Vyvanse, stimulant for ADHD)
Narrow Therapeutic Index: No
Precautions: Avoid during pregnancy; monitor potassium and kidney labs; do not combine with ARBs (-sartans)
Routes: Oral
Easily Replaceable? Yes – several equivalent "-prils" are available

Sample Test Questions:
Q: What side effect often leads to switching to an Angiotensin II receptor blocker (ARB)?
A: Dry cough
Q: Why should ACE inhibitors and ARBs be avoided in pregnancy?
A: Birth defects

#4 Levothyroxine (SYNTHROID, T4 thyroid hormone)

lee-voh-thy-ROX-een (SIN-throyd)

Common Uses: Hypothyroidism (low thyroid)

Mascot: "Four I'd monster" – levothyroxine contains 4 iodine (I) atoms

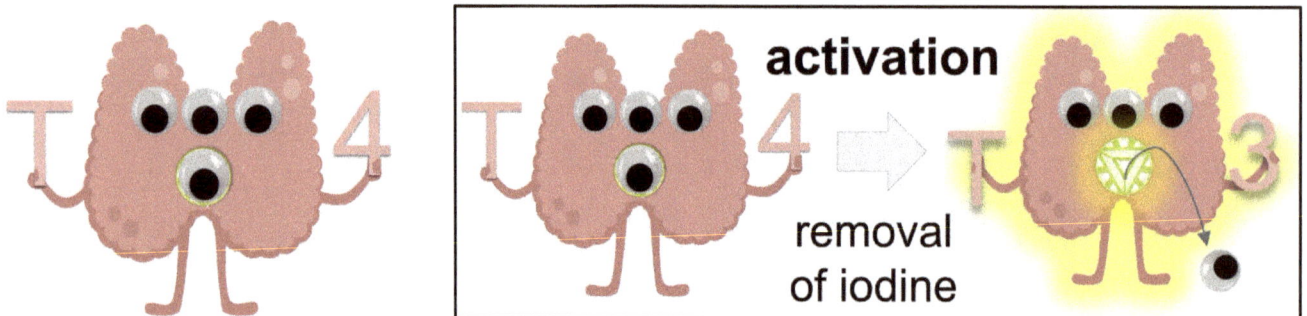

activation
removal
of iodine

Alternate Mnemonics:

❖ "Levo- Leaves you waiting" – works slower than T3

❖ "Levo-lifts sluggish thyroids"

❖ "Synthroid = synthetic thyroid"

❖ "Leave it to levo- to alleviate low thyroid

Drug Class: Hormone replacement: Thyroid hormone: T4

Similar Drugs: Liothyronine = T3 (#204), Armour Thyroid = desiccated T4 + T3 (#137) **Comparisons:** Works slower but lasts longer than liothyronine (T3)

Controlled Substance: ✅ Not controlled

High-Alert Risk: ⚠️ ⚠️ Requires careful dosing – too much can cause fast heartbeat or weight loss; do not use as a weight-loss medication

Major Side Effects: Fast heart rate, anxiety, weight loss (if overdosed)

Look-Alike/Sound-Alike: Lanoxin, liothyronine

Narrow Therapeutic Index: Yes

Precautions: Take on empty stomach; don't switch brands without checking

Routes: Oral, IV

Easily Replaceable? No – the body converts T4 to T3. Giving T3 (liothyronine) directly bypasses this natural control and can cause temporary hyperthyroid states.

Also: Must be taken 30–60 minutes before food for proper absorption

Sample Test Questions:

Q: What organ does levothyroxine replace hormones for?

A: Thyroid

Q: What is a major danger of taking too much levothyroxine?

A: Fast heart rate (tachycardia) or weight loss

Q: Should levothyroxine be taken with food?

A: No – take on an empty stomach

#5 Amlodipine (NORVASC)

am-LOH-duh-peen (NOR-vask)
Common Uses: High blood pressure, chest pain (angina)
Mascot: "I am loading Nora's vasculature"

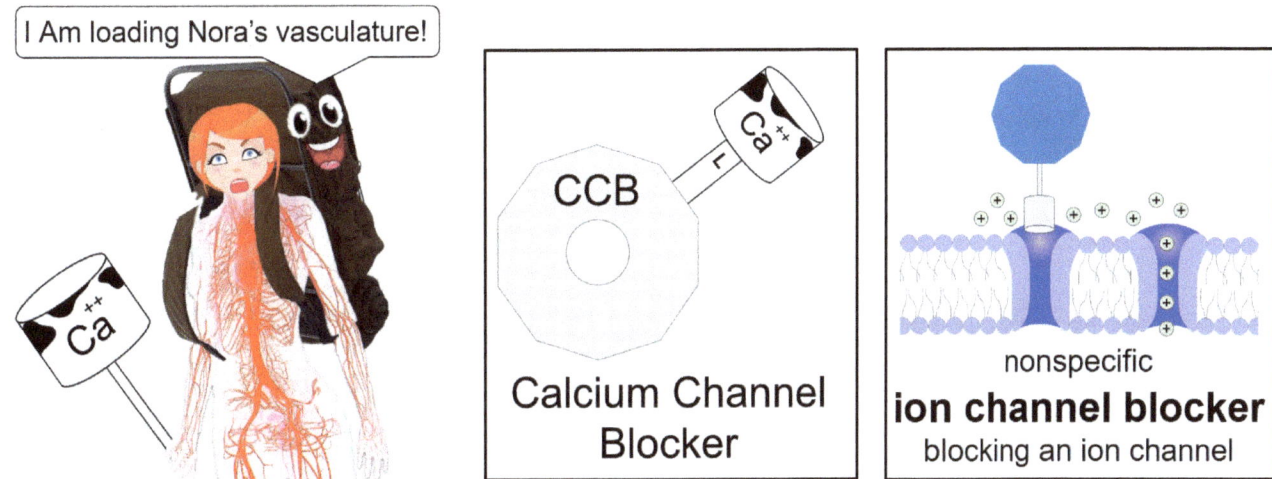

Alternate Mnemonics:

❖ "Ample dilation = lower pressure." – dilates arterioles to lower blood pressure (BP)

❖ "I Am lowering Nora's BP"

❖ "Amlow, dipping BP"

❖ "Norvasc = normalizing vascular squeeze"

Drug Class: Blood pressure medication: Calcium channel blocker
Similar Drugs: Nifedipine (#151)
Comparisons: Longer-acting and better tolerated than nifedipine
High-Alert Risk: ✅ Not high alert
Major Side Effects: Swelling in legs (edema), lightheadedness due to BP decrease
Look-Alike/Sound-Alike: Amantadine
Narrow Therapeutic Index: No
Precautions: Watch for swelling or low blood pressure
Routes: Oral
Easily Replaceable? Yes – other calcium channel blockers ("-dipines") may be used
Also: May take 7–10 days for full effect on blood pressure

Sample Test Questions:
Q: What side effect may cause leg swelling in patients on amlodipine?
A: Peripheral edema
Q: How long may it take for amlodipine to fully lower blood pressure?
A: 7 to 10 days

#6 Metoprolol (LOPRESSOR, TOPROL XL)

meh-TOE-pro-lol (LOH-press-or, TOH-prol)
Common Uses: High blood pressure, heart failure, post-heart attack
Mascot: "Low-pressure Meet-up"

➤ Beta blockers end in -olol and their mascots wear an "LOL" hat

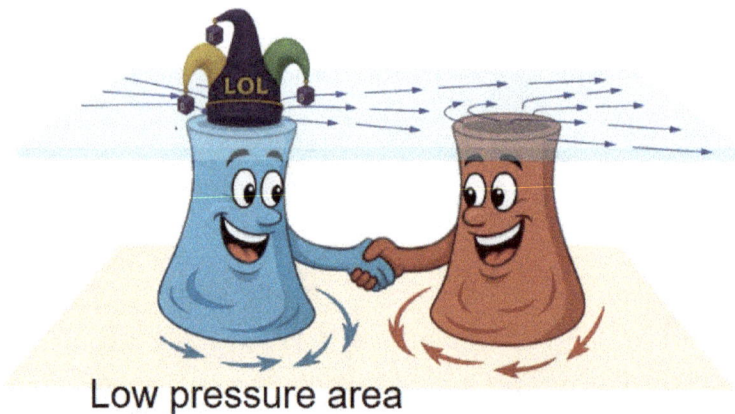

Low pressure area

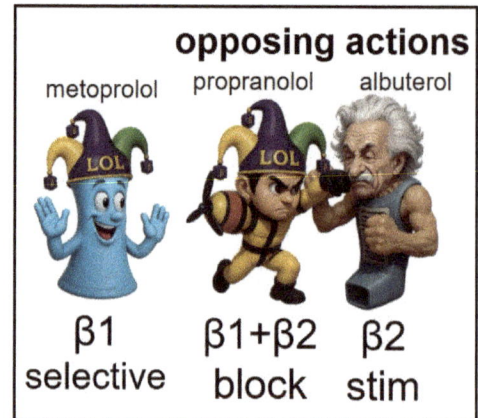

opposing actions

metoprolol — propranolol — albuterol

β1 selective — β1+β2 block — β2 stim

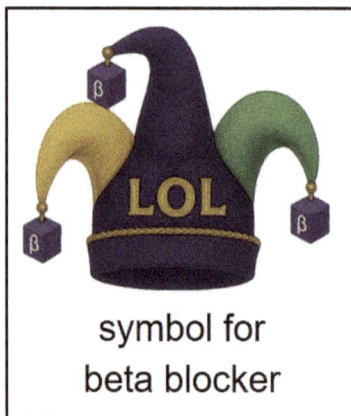

symbol for beta blocker

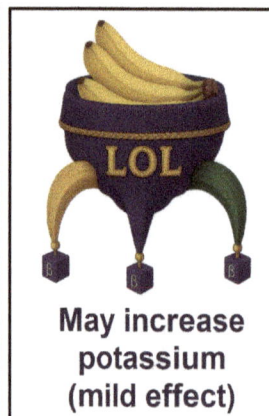

May increase potassium (mild effect)

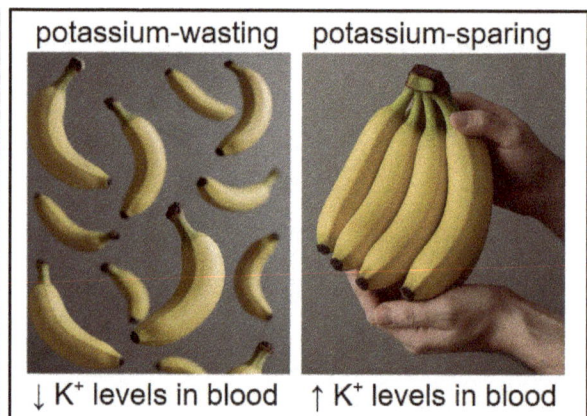

potassium-wasting — potassium-sparing

↓ K⁺ levels in blood — ↑ K⁺ levels in blood

Alternate Mnemonics:

❖ "Metoprolol taps the brakes on BP"

❖ "Metoprolol slows heart rate, LOL"

❖ "Metoprolol = mellowed pulse"

❖ "Metoprolol tartrate slows your heart rate"

❖ "Toprol tames tachy" – tachycardia = fast heart rate

❖ *Beta Blockers* song available on YouTube, Spotify, etc

Drug Class: Blood pressure and heart medication: Beta blocker (β1 selective)
Similar Drugs: Atenolol (#63), Carvedilol (#34), Propranolol (#77), Nebivolol (#173)
Comparisons: Unlike beta blockers acting on β1 and β2 receptors, metoprolol is selective for β1, so it is less likely to cause bronchospasm than non-selective beta blockers

➤ β1 is in heart, β2 is in lungs – "you have 1 heart, 2 lungs"

CARDIOSELECTIVE β BLOCKERS (β1)
➤ unlikely to cause bronchospasm

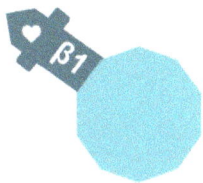

Cross blood-brain barrier (BBB):
❖ **bisoprolol**
❖ **metoprolol**
❖ **nebivolol**
➤ also nitric oxide

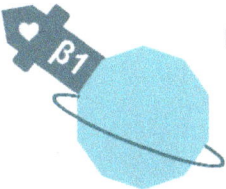

Do not cross BBB:
❖ **atenolol**
❖ **esmolol**

NONSELECTIVE β BLOCKERS (β1 + β2)
➤ avoid in moderate/severe asthma

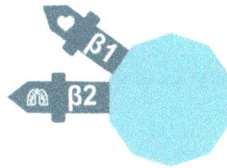

Cross blood-brain barrier (BBB):
❖ **propranolol**
❖ **pindolol**
❖ **timolol**
❖ **carvedilol**
➤ also α1 block

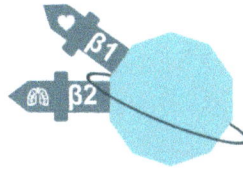

Do not cross BBB:
❖ **nadolol**
❖ **sotalol**
➤ other effects
❖ **labetalol**
➤ also α1 block

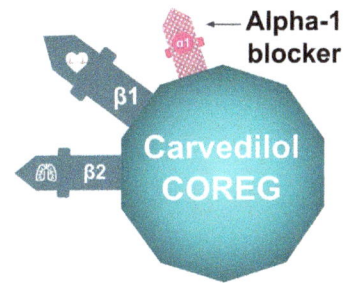

← Alpha-1 blocker

Carvedilol COREG

BETA RECEPTOR AGONISTS
➤ epinephrine and norepinephrine receptor stimulators

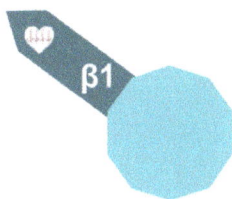

β1 AGONISTS
❖ **dobutamine**
➤ ↑ heart rate to treat acute heart failure

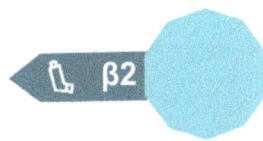

β2 AGONIST INHALERS
❖ **albuterol**
❖ **levalbuterol**
❖ **salmeterol**
❖ **vilanterol**

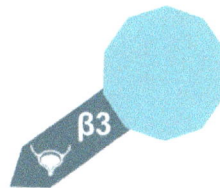

β3 AGONISTS FOR OVERACTIVE BLADDER
❖ **mirabegron**
❖ **vibegron**

Formulations:
➤ Lopressor = regular form, immediate release metoprolol <u>tartrate</u>, short-acting (twice daily)
➤ Toprol XL = extended release metoprolol <u>succinate</u> (once daily)

High-Alert Risk: ✅ Not high alert, although heart rate and BP may be too low if the dose is too high

Major Side Effects: Slow heart rate, tiredness, lightheadedness

Look-Alike/Sound-Alike: Metoclopramide

Narrow Therapeutic Index: No

Precautions: Don't stop suddenly; taper slowly

Routes: Oral, IV

Easily Replaceable? Yes – several beta blockers ("-olols") are available

Sample Test Questions:

Q: What is the difference between Lopressor and Toprol XL?

A: Lopressor is short-acting (tartrate), Toprol XL is extended-release (succinate)

Q: What drug class has the opposite effect of beta blockers?

A: Beta agonists, including albuterol (#7)

#7 Albuterol (VENTOLIN HFA)

al-BYOO-ter-ol (VEN-toe-lin)
Common Uses: Rescue inhaler for asthma and COPD wheezing or shortness of breath
Mascot: "Albert, all Ventilated"

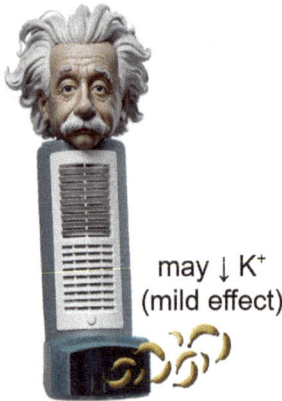

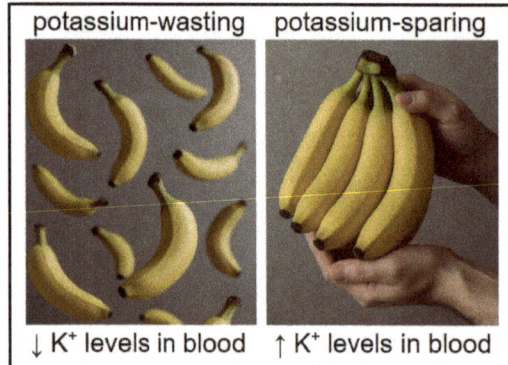

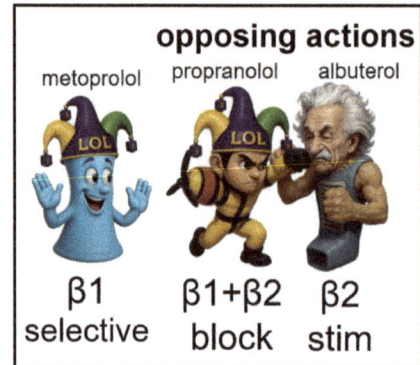

may ↓ K^+
(mild effect)

potassium-wasting	potassium-sparing
↓ K^+ levels in blood	↑ K^+ levels in blood

opposing actions

metoprolol	propranolol	albuterol
β1 selective	β1+β2 block	β2 stim

Alternate Mnemonics:

❖ "Albuterol = air booster"

❖ "Ventolin vents the lungs"

❖ "ProAir provides air"

Trade Names: VENTOLIN HFA, PROAIR HFA, PROVENTIL HFA
Drug Class: Bronchodilator: Short-Acting Beta-2 Agonist (SABA)
Similar Drugs: Levalbuterol (SABA)
Comparisons: Levalbuterol (left-handed molecule) is the "pure" form with fewer side effects
➤ Long-acting β2 agonists (LABAs) include Salmeterol (#59) and Formoterol (#83)
High-Alert Risk: ✅ Not high alert
Major Side Effects: Tremor, nervousness, rapid heart rate, low potassium if heavy use
Look-Alike/Sound-Alike: Albendazole, labetalol
Narrow Therapeutic Index: No
Routes: Metered dose inhaler (MDI), nebulizer (converts liquid to mist over several minutes)

Easily Replaceable? Yes – other drugs in this class are comparable

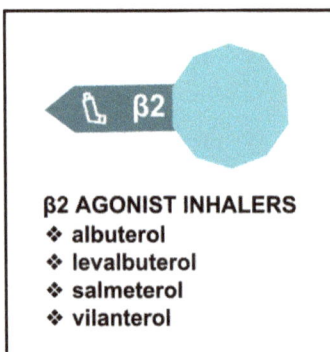

β2

β2 AGONIST INHALERS
❖ albuterol
❖ levalbuterol
❖ salmeterol
❖ vilanterol

Sample Test Questions:
Q: What is a common side effect of albuterol?
A: Tremor or tachycardia
Q: What warning sign may indicate albuterol overuse?
A: Needing the inhaler more than twice per week
Q: What is a rare but serious adverse effect of albuterol?
A: Paradoxical bronchospasm

#8 Losartan (Cozaar)

loh-SAR-tan (COH-zar)

Common Uses: High blood pressure, kidney protection in diabetes

Mascot: "Cozier Lord sa(r)tan"

➤ Sartan mascots are devils – the "Satans"

➤ He is wearing a modified Arby's logo because losartan is an ARB

➤ Sartans may elevate potassium levels (represented by bananas)

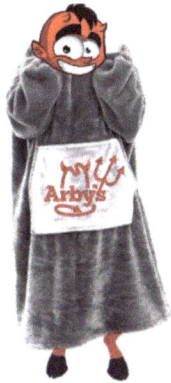

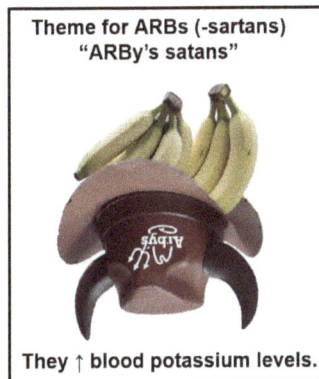

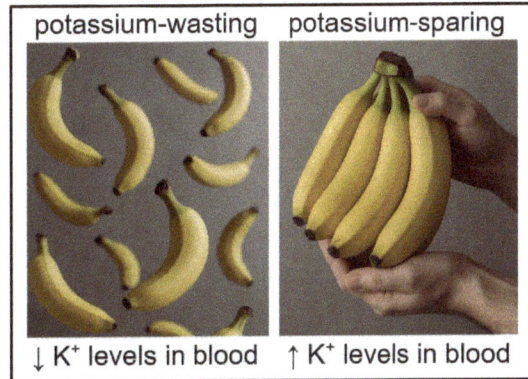

Theme for ARBs (-sartans)
"ARBy's satans"

They ↑ blood potassium levels.

potassium-wasting | potassium-sparing
↓ K+ levels in blood | ↑ K+ levels in blood

Alternate Mnemonics:

❖ "Low pressure with Losartan"

❖ "Losartan loosens the squeeze"

Drug Class: Antihypertensive (blood pressure-lowering medication): Angiotensin II Receptor Blocker (ARB) – "Sartan"

Similar Drugs (Top 300): Valsartan (#117), Olmesartan (#97), Losartan/HCTZ (#75) **Comparisons:** Similar to ACE inhibitors but causes less cough

High-Alert Risk: ✅ Not high alert

Major Side Effects: Dizziness, high potassium

Look-Alike/Sound-Alike: Lisinopril

Narrow Therapeutic Index: No

Precautions: Avoid in pregnancy; monitor potassium and kidney function

Routes: Oral

Easily Substituted? Yes – several equivalent "sartans" are available

Also: Often combined with HCTZ in a single daily tablet

Sample Test Questions:

Q: What type of blood pressure drug is losartan?

A: ARB (Angiotensin II Receptor Blocker)

Q: Why is losartan often chosen over ACE inhibitors?

A: It causes less cough

Q: What lab should be monitored during losartan use?

A: Potassium

#9 Omeprazole (PRILOSEC)

oh-MEP-ruh-zole (PRY-lo-sec)

Common Uses: Ulcers (sores or breaks in the lining of the stomach or intestines), gastroesophageal reflux disease (GERD)

Mascot: "Ome pries Loose – Oh my!"

➤ A stomach named Ome, "prying loose" a proton (H^+) pump

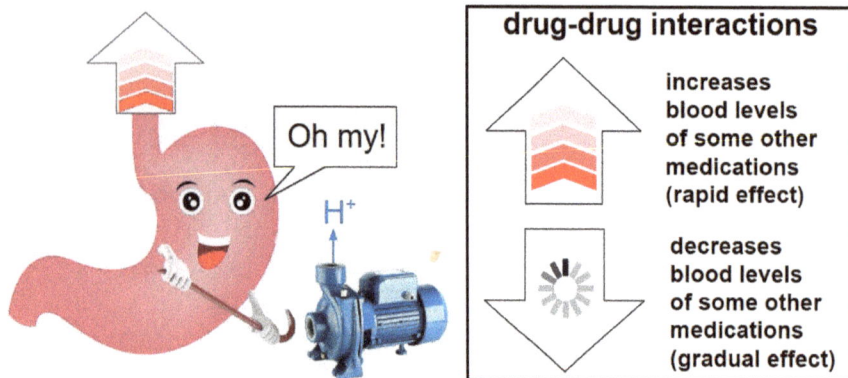

Alternate Mnemonics:

❖ "Ome, prays it stops the burn"

❖ "OTC Ome works overtime on ulcers" (OTC = over-the-counter without prescription)

Drug Class: Stomach acid reducer: Proton pump inhibitor (PPI)

Similar Drugs: Pantoprazole (#16), Esomeprazole (#122), Lansoprazole (#224)

Comparisons: Pantoprazole (prescription-only) is preferred over omeprazole (OTC and Rx) because pantoprazole has fewer drug interactions and more predictable absorption

High-Alert Risk: ⚠ Potential for drug-drug interactions

Major Side Effects: Diarrhea, low magnesium or vitamin B12, osteoporosis (bone thinning)

Look-Alike/Sound-Alike: Esomeprazole (#122)

Narrow Therapeutic Index: No

Precautions: Avoid unnecessary long-term use; taper to prevent rebound acid

Routes: Oral

Easily Replaceable? Yes – other PPIs ("-prazoles") often used

Also: Best taken 30–60 minutes before the first meal of the day; Omeprazole increases levels of some drugs including the blood thinner clopidogrel (Plavix) and the antidepressant escitalopram (Lexapro)

Sample Test Questions:

Q: When should omeprazole be taken?

A: 30–60 minutes before breakfast

Q: What risk is linked to long-term use of omeprazole?

A: Bone fractures – applicable to all proton pump inhibitors, due to decreased bone strength

#10 Gabapentin (NEURONTIN)

GAB-a-pen-tin (NUR-on-tin)
Common Uses: Nerve pain, seizures, anxiety, restless legs syndrome
Mascot: "Gabba pen tin" = "Neuron tin"

➤ Pens shaped like neurons with heads of Yo Gabba Gabba characters

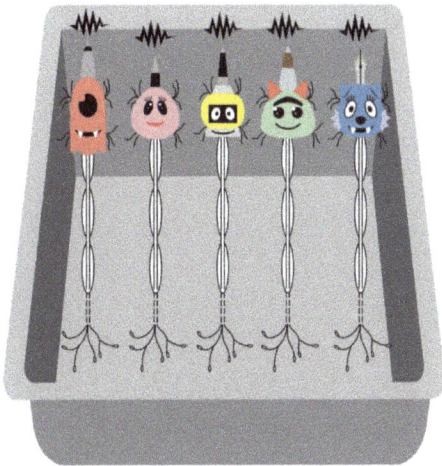

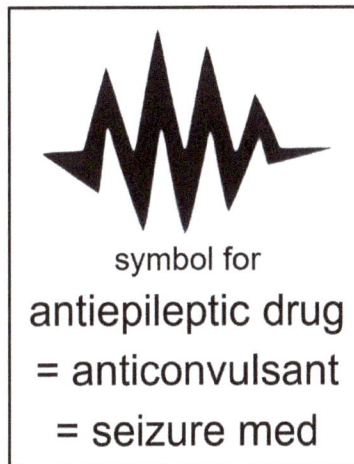

symbol for
antiepileptic drug
= anticonvulsant
= seizure med

Alternate Mnemonics:

❖ "Neu-rotten for rotten nerves"

❖ "Gabapentin stops Gabby nerves from tingling" (Gabby = just a made-up word)

Drug Class: Antiepileptic (anti-seizure medication): GABA analog / gabapentinoid
Similar Drugs: Pregabalin (#91)
Comparisons: Pregabalin, the other gabapentinoid, is a Schedule V controlled substance with stronger anti-anxiety effect; Gabapentin is less likely to cause swelling in legs (edema) than pregabalin
Controlled Substance: ✅ Not controlled federally ⚠️ Schedule V in some states
High-Alert Risk: ⚠️ Mild – may be misused, especially with opioids
Major Side Effects: Sleepiness, lightheadedness, swelling in legs (edema)
Narrow Therapeutic Index: No – less efficiently absorbed at higher doses
Precautions: Lower dose in kidney problems; taper slowly to stop

➤ Seizure is possible if any anti-seizure medication is stopped without tapering

Routes: Oral
Easily Replaceable? Partially – pregabalin is similar but not identical
Also: Often dosed 3 times per day for full effect

Sample Test Questions:
Q: What is a major side effect of gabapentin?
A: Sleepiness
Q: Can gabapentin be stopped suddenly?
A: No – any anti-seizure medication should be tapered gradually

#11 Sertraline (ZOLOFT)

SUR-truh-leen (ZOH-loft)

Common Uses: Depression, anxiety, obsessive-compulsive disorder (OCD), post-traumatic stress disorder (PTSD)

Mascot: "So soft on the Shirt line"

- ➤ The "Baby on Board" shirt refers to sertraline as the preferred antidepressant during pregnancy
- ➤ "So soft" refers to possible side effects of diarrhea and erectile dysfunction

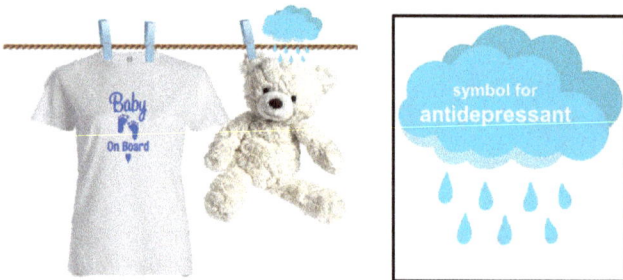

Alternate Mnemonics:

- ❖ "Certainly tonin' your mood with serotonin"
- ❖ If they've tried several antidepressants, they've almost "certainly tried" sertraline
- ❖ "Mood, so lofty"
- ❖ "Sertraline keeps sadness in line"

Drug Class: Antidepressant: Selective Serotonin Reuptake Inhibitor (SSRI)

Similar Drugs: Escitalopram (#15), Fluoxetine (#22), Citalopram (#40), Paroxetine (#92)

Comparisons: Fewer drug-drug interactions than fluoxetine or paroxetine

High-Alert Risk: ✅ Not high alert, although warning of suicidal thoughts in patients under age 25 – applicable to all antidepressants

     ➤ Serotonin toxicity – dangerous if combined with a monoamine oxidase inhibitor (MAOI) – phenelzine, tranylcypromine, isocarboxazid, selegiline, linezolid, or methylene blue

Major Side Effects: Nausea, insomnia, diarrhea, sexual dysfunction, serotonin withdrawal symptoms when stopping

Look-Alike/Sound-Alike: Seroquel

Narrow Therapeutic Index: ✅ No – wide therapeutic index; <1/10,000 single-drug overdose fatality risk

Precautions: Takes weeks to work; do not stop suddenly to avoid unpleasant serotonin withdrawal

Routes: Oral

Easily Replaceable? Partially – SSRIs are similar, but psychiatric meds often require individualization a

Sample Test Questions:

Q: How long may it take for sertraline to show benefit?

A: Several weeks – applicable to all SSRIs

Q: What side effect most often leads patients to quit taking sertraline?

A: Sexual dysfunction – applicable to all SSRIs

#12 Hydrochlorothiazide (MICROZIDE)

HYE-droe-KLOR-oh-THY-a-zide (MY-croh-zide)
Common Uses: High blood pressure, fluid retention
Standard Abbreviation: HCTZ
Mascot: "Micro Hydrant, tie-dyed"

➤ Thiazide diuretics wear a tie-dyed die

➤ The mascot is micro-sized, 2.5 cm according to the ruler

potassium-wasting	potassium-sparing
↓ K⁺ levels in blood	↑ K⁺ levels in blood

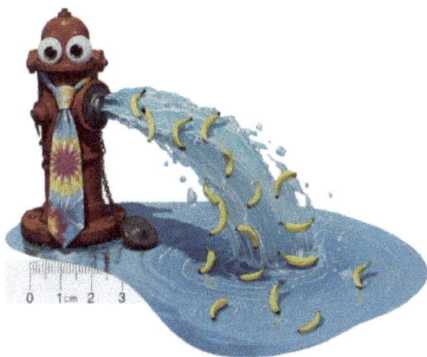

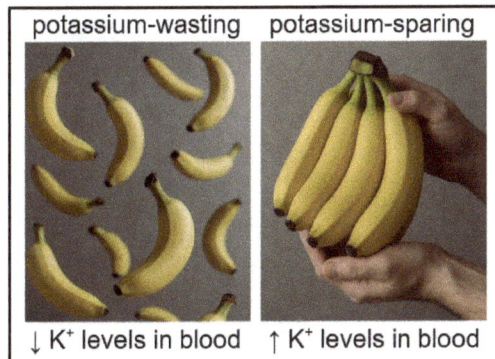

Alternate mnemonics:

❖ "Hydro clears water, drops pressure" – diuretics increase urination and are called "water pills" informally

❖ "Hydrochlorothiazide = Hydro + Chloride exits" (along with sodium and potassium)

❖ "HCTZ helps clear the tank"

❖ "Microzide = micro pee slide"

Drug Class: Blood pressure medication: Diuretic: Thiazide diuretic (potassium-wasting)
Similar Drugs: Chlorthalidone (#108), HCTZ/lisinopril combo (#53), HCTZ/losartan combo (#75)
Comparisons: Less potent and shorter acting than chlorthalidone
High-Alert Risk: ✅ Not high alert
Major Side Effects: Low potassium, dizziness, frequent urination
Look-Alike/Sound-Alike: Hydrocodone
Narrow Therapeutic Index: No
Precautions: Monitor electrolytes; may increase blood sugar or uric acid
Routes: Oral
Easily Replaceable? Yes – several thiazide-type diuretics available
Also: Best taken in the morning to avoid nighttime urination

Sample Test Questions:
Q: What electrolyte can be lost when taking HCTZ?
A: Potassium
Q: HCTZ should be taken in the morning due to what side effect that affects sleep?
A: Frequent urination

#13 Rosuvastatin (CRESTOR)

roh-SOO-vuh-stat-in (CRES-tor)
Common Uses: High cholesterol
Mascot: "Cresty Roosta-statin"

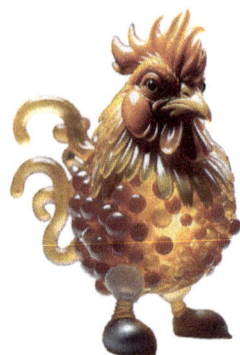

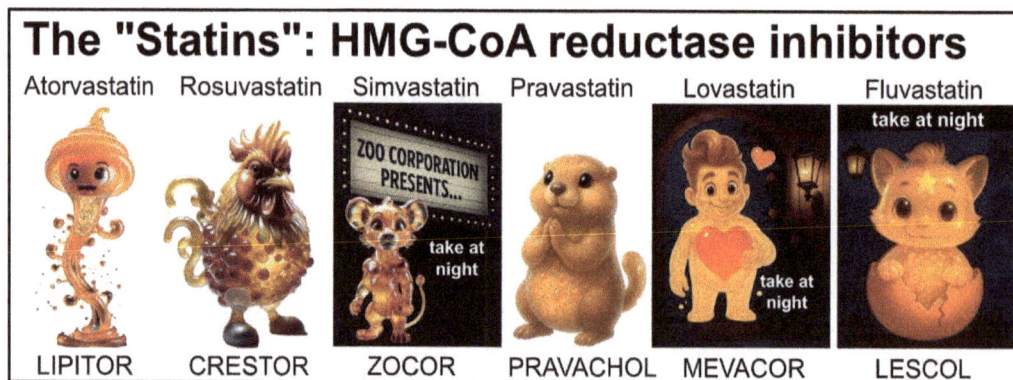

The "Statins": HMG-CoA reductase inhibitors

Atorvastatin	Rosuvastatin	Simvastatin	Pravastatin	Lovastatin	Fluvastatin
LIPITOR	CRESTOR	ZOCOR	PRAVACHOL	MEVACOR	LESCOL

Alternate Mnemonics:

❖ "Stat-in for fat-in your arteries"
❖ "Rose to the top for cholesterol drop"
❖ "Rosu is robust among statins"
❖ "Crestor = crest of potency"
❖ "Rosuvastatin rises above LDL"
❖ "Rosuvastatin = strong, steady statin"
❖ "Rosu clears the cholesterol runway"

Drug Class: Cholesterol-lowering: Statin (HMG-CoA reductase inhibitor)
Similar Drugs: Atorvastatin (#1), Simvastatin (#19), Pravastatin (#37), Lovastatin (#111)
Comparisons: More potent than most statins; fewer drug interactions
High-Alert Risk: ✅ Not high alert
Major Side Effects: Muscle pain, liver problems
Look-Alike/Sound-Alike: Rivastigmine
Narrow Therapeutic Index: No
Precautions: Avoid in liver disease; check muscle symptoms
Routes: Oral
Easily Replaceable? Yes – other statins may be used
Also: May be taken any time of day, with or without food

Sample Test Questions:
Q: What is a major organ monitored during statin use?
A: Liver
Q: What symptom should be reported when on any HMG-CoA reductase inhibitor?
A: Muscle pain, which is a sign of rhabdomyolysis (muscle breakdown)

#14 Mixed Amphetamine Salts (ADDERALL)

AM-fet-uh-meen (ADD-er-all)
Common Uses: ADHD, narcolepsy
Mascot: "Amp to Add it all"

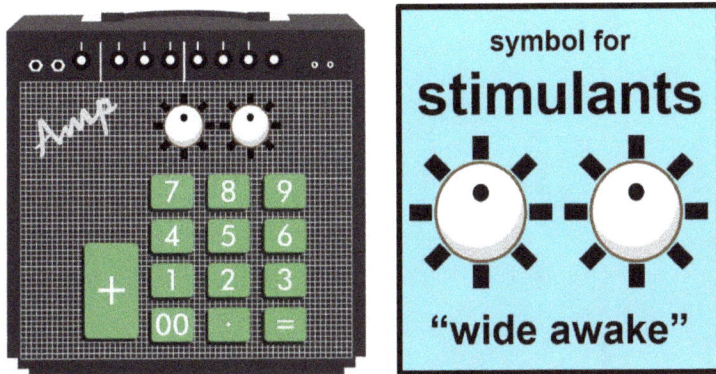

Alternate Mnemonics:
- ❖ "Amphetamine adds alertness"
- ❖ "Adderall for all ADD" (Attention Deficit Disorder)
- ❖ "Adderall adds attention"

Drug Class: ADHD medication: CNS stimulant: Amphetamine
Similar Drugs: Methylphenidate (#32), Lisdexamfetamine (#69), Dexmethylphenidate (#109)
Comparisons: Longer acting than dextroamphetamine alone
Controlled Substance: ⚠ ⚠ ⚠ C-II
> ► C-II controlled substances (opioids, stimulants) and more strictly controlled than C-IV (benzos)

High-Alert Risk: ⚠ ⚠ Controlled due to misuse/abuse risk
Major Side Effects: Insomnia, fast heart rate, appetite loss
Look-Alike/Sound-Alike: Atomoxetine
Narrow Therapeutic Index: No
Precautions: Risk of dependence; avoid late-day dosing
Routes: Oral
Easily Replaceable? Partially – other stimulants used but not identical
Also: Not highly addictive, but potentially abusable – methamphetamine-like euphoria at high doses

Sample Test Questions:
Q: What class of controlled substance is Adderall?
A: Schedule II (C-II)
Q: What is a common cardiovascular side effect of amphetamines?
A: Fast heart rate (tachycardia)
Q: Why should Adderall be taken early in the day?
A: To avoid insomnia

#15 Escitalopram (LEXAPRO)

ES-sih-TAL-oh-pram (LEX-uh-pro)
Common Uses: Depression, anxiety
Mascot: "Lexus Pram" – pram is the British word for baby carriage

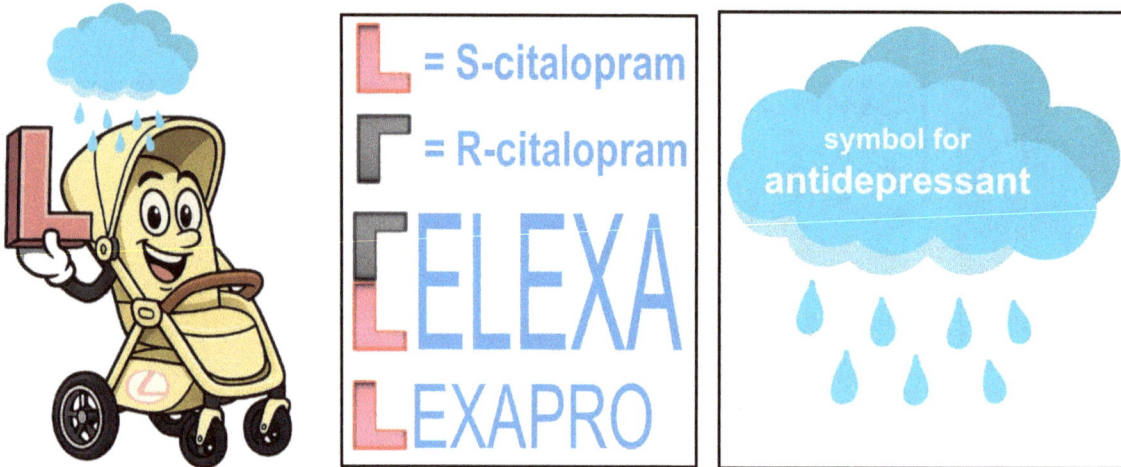

L = S-citalopram
Г = R-citalopram
CELEXA
LEXAPRO

symbol for **antidepressant**

Alternate Mnemonics:
- ❖ "Escitalopram = escape depression and anxiety"
- ❖ "S-citalopram = simplified serotonin support" – It's the "pure" form of citalopram (Celexa)

Drug Class: Antidepressant: SSRI (Selective Serotonin Reuptake Inhibitor)
Similar SSRIs: Sertraline (#11), Fluoxetine (#22), Citalopram (#40), Paroxetine (#92)
Comparisons: Well tolerated; fewer side effects than older SSRIs
Controlled Substance: ✅ Not controlled
High-Alert Risk: ✅ Not high alert, although warning of suicidal thoughts in patients under age 25 – applicable to all antidepressants
➤ Serotonin toxicity – dangerous if combined with a monoamine oxidase inhibitor (MAOI) – phenelzine, tranylcypromine, isocarboxazid, selegiline, linezolid, or methylene blue
Major Side Effects: Nausea, headache, sexual dysfunction, insomnia
Look-Alike/Sound-Alike: Citalopram
Narrow Therapeutic Index: No
Precautions: Taper slowly to avoid withdrawal symptoms
Routes: Oral
Easily Replaceable? Partially – SSRIs are similar, but psychiatric medications often require trial and error

Sample Test Questions:
Q: What neurotransmitter does escitalopram affect?
A: Serotonin
Q: How should escitalopram be discontinued?
A: Slowly tapered to avoid withdrawal symptoms

#16 Pantoprazole (PROTONIX)

pan-TOH-pruh-zole (PRO-tuh-nix)
Common Uses: Gastroesophageal reflux disease (GERD), ulcers, erosive esophagitis
Mascot: "Proton Pants"

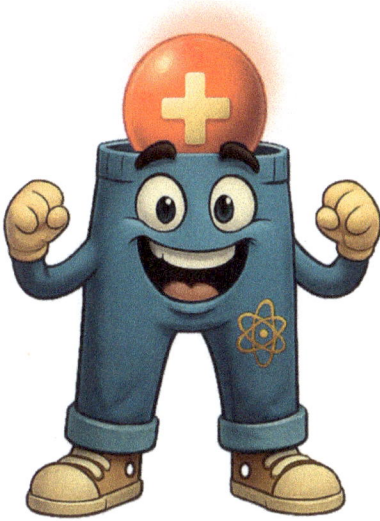

Alternate Mnemonics:

❖ "Pantoprazole, the Pro PPI" (prescription only)

❖ "Pants nix protons"

❖ "Pro-tonix: protects from protonic fire" – protons (H^+) are acidic

Drug Class: Acid reducer: Proton pump inhibitor (PPI)
Similar PPIs: Omeprazole (#9), Esomeprazole (#122), Lansoprazole (#224)
Comparisons: Fewer drug-drug interactions than omeprazole
High-Alert Risk: ✅ Not high alert
Major Side Effects: Low magnesium, diarrhea, B12 deficiency
Look-Alike/Sound-Alike: Propranolol
Narrow Therapeutic Index: No
Precautions: Long-term use may lead to bone loss and C. difficile infection
Routes: Oral, IV
Easily Replaceable? Yes – other PPIs available

Sample Test Questions:
Q: What is the mechanism of action of pantoprazole?
A: It blocks proton pumps to reduce stomach acid production
Q: What long-term risk is associated with pantoprazole use?
A: Osteoporosis or bone fracture
Q: What vitamin may be deficient with long-term PPI use?
A: Vitamin B12

#17 Montelukast (SINGULAIR)

mon-TELL-oo-kast (SING-yoo-lair)

Common Uses: Asthma prevention, allergic rhinitis

Mascot: "Monte's leukotriene Singularity"

➤ The Singularity is a hypothetical point where AI surpasses or merges with human intelligence

➤ Leukotrienes are chemicals made by your immune system that cause inflammation

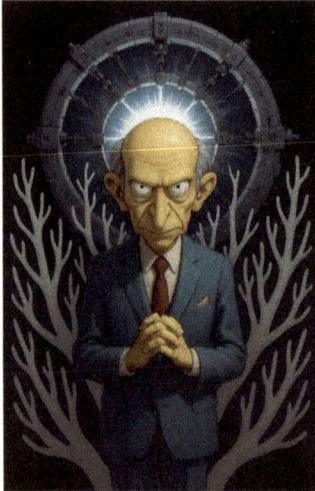

Alternate Mnemonics:

❖ "Monte blocks leukotrienes in the airways"

❖ "Mount the airway defense against asthma"

❖ "Single-air"

Drug Class: Asthma/allergy controller: Leukotriene receptor antagonist

Similar Drugs: None in same class

Comparisons: A pill, not an inhaler; Used for prevention, not acute attacks

High-Alert Risk: ✅ Not high alert

Major Side Effects: Headache, abdominal pain, mood changes

Look-Alike/Sound-Alike: Motrin

Narrow Therapeutic Index: No

Precautions: Not a rescue medication; does not treat acute attacks

➤ Warning for possible neuropsychiatric effects including suicidal thoughts

Routes: Oral

Easily Replaceable? No – unique drug class

Sample Test Questions:

Q: Is montelukast used for quick relief of asthma? A:

No – it is used for prevention

Q: What warning was added to montelukast in 2020?

A: Risk of mental health/mood changes

#18 Trazodone (DESYREL)

TRAZ-oh-doan (DEZ-uh-rel)

Common Uses: Insomnia (off-label, 50–150 mg), depression (the FDA-approved indication, although trazodone is rarely prescribed at the antidepressant dose of 200–600 mg)

Mascot: "Desy's Trays o' bone"

➤ Bones for "boner" – rare risk of priapism (prolonged erection)

➤ The polka dots on pink pattern mean it's an alpha-1 blocker – orthostatic hypotension (low blood pressure when standing up) and syncope (fainting) is possible – "hit the floor"

➤ Alpha-1 block with this medication is an off-target effect, unrelated to its antidepressant effect

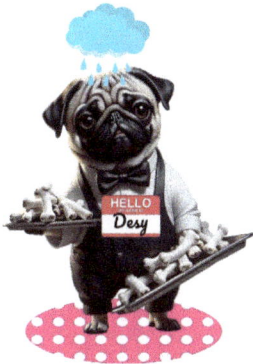

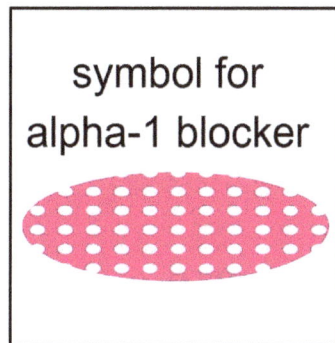

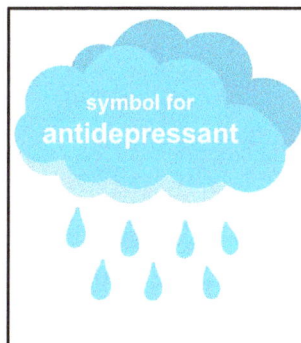

Alternate Mnemonics:

❖ "Trazzzz for sleep"

❖ "Traz-o-bone" (rare risk of priapism)

❖ "Trazodone = drowsy zone"

Drug Class: Antidepressant: Serotonin modulator / Atypical antidepressant

Similar Drugs: Mirtazapine (#105)

Comparisons: While trazodone is usually just for sleep, mirtazapine (Remeron) is usually prescribed for depression with insomnia; Mirtazapine causes weight gain, while trazodone does not

Controlled Substance: ✅ Not controlled

High-Alert Risk: ✅ Not high alert

Major Side Effects: Sedation, dizziness, dry mouth, priapism (rare)

Look-Alike/Sound-Alike: Tramadol

Narrow Therapeutic Index: No

Precautions: Risk of fall in elderly

Routes: Oral

Sample Test Questions:

Q: What is the most common use for trazodone?

A: Sleep aid

Q: What serious but rare side effect should male patients be warned about?

A: Priapism – seek immediate medical care if erection lasts more than 4 hours

#19 Simvastatin (ZOCOR)

SIM-vuh-stat-in (ZOH-cor)
Common Uses: High cholesterol
Mascot: "Zoo Corp's Simba-statin"

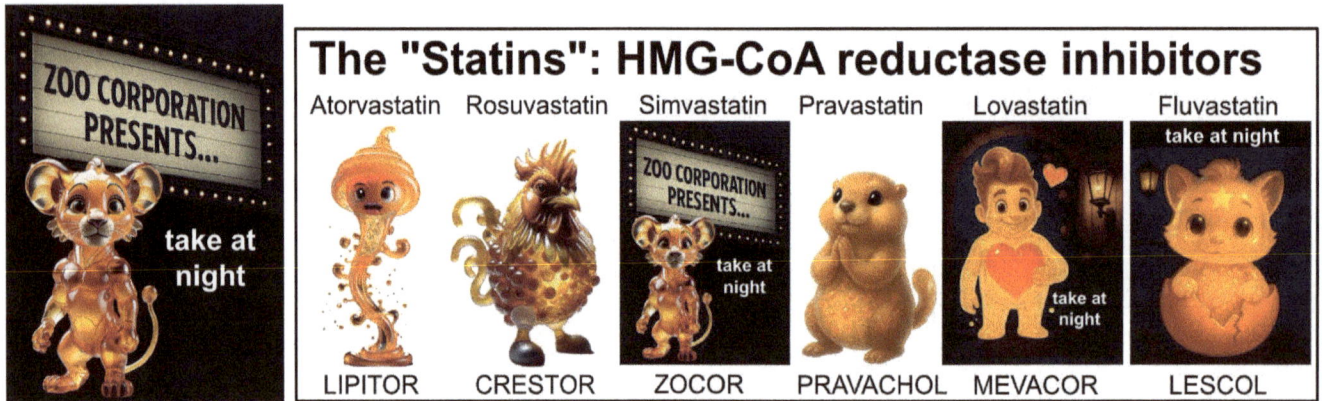

The "Statins": HMG-CoA reductase inhibitors

Atorvastatin — LIPITOR
Rosuvastatin — CRESTOR
Simvastatin — ZOCOR (take at night)
Pravastatin — PRAVACHOL
Lovastatin — MEVACOR (take at night)
Fluvastatin — LESCOL (take at night)

Alternate Mnemonics:

❖ "Simmer down that LDL" – Low density lipoproteins (LDL) = bad cholesterol

❖ "Simvastatin = simpler, older statin"

❖ "Zocor zaps cholesterol"

Drug Class: Cholesterol-lowering: HMG-CoA reductase inhibitor (Statin)
Similar Statins: Atorvastatin (#1), Rosuvastatin (#13), Pravastatin (#37), Lovastatin (#111)
Comparisons: More drug interactions than atorvastatin; less potent
High-Alert Risk: ✅ Not high alert
Major Side Effects: Muscle pain, liver enzyme elevation
Look-Alike/Sound-Alike: Sinequan
Narrow Therapeutic Index: No
Precautions: Avoid grapefruit – grapefruit increases levels of many medications, including simvastatin
Routes: Oral
Easily Replaceable? Yes – other statins available

Sample Test Questions:
Q: When should simvastatin be taken?
A: At bedtime
Q: What fruit should be avoided with simvastatin?
A: Grapefruit
Q: What serious muscle-related condition may occur with statins?
A: Rhabdomyolysis (muscle breakdown)

#20 Tamsulosin (FLOMAX)

tam-SOO-loh-sin (FLOH-max)

Common Uses: Benign prostatic hyperplasia (BPH, enlarged prostate)

Mascot: "Tiramisu losin' Flow maximizer"

➤ The polka dots on pink pattern mean it's an alpha-1 blocker – orthostatic hypotension (low blood pressure when standing) and syncope (fainting) is possible – "hit the floor"

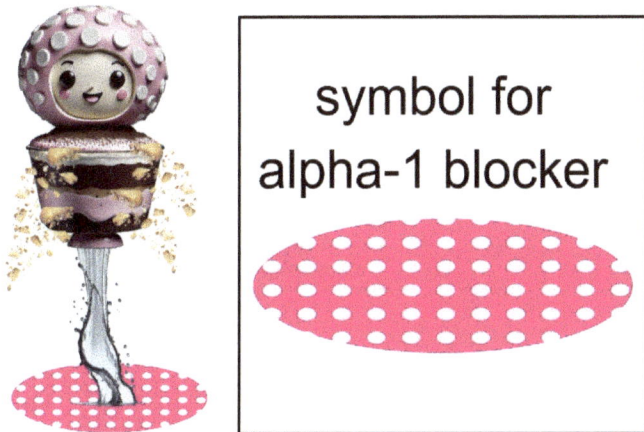

symbol for alpha-1 blocker

Alternate Mnemonics:

❖ "Flo-max = maximizes flow"

❖ "Tamsu-low-sin = lowers pressure in prostate"

❖ "Flomax: flows through the prostate gate"

Drug Class: BPH treatment: Alpha-1 blocker

Similar Drugs: Doxazosin (#180)

Comparisons: More selective for the prostate than older alpha-blockers

Controlled Substance: ✅ Not controlled

High-Alert Risk: ✅ Not high alert

Major Side Effects: Dizziness, low blood pressure

Look-Alike/Sound-Alike: Tamiflu

Narrow Therapeutic Index: No

Precautions: Take 30 minutes after the same meal each day; May cause orthostatic hypotension (low blood pressure upon standing) or fainting

Routes: Oral

Easily Replaceable? Yes – other alpha-blockers available but less prostate-selective

Sample Test Questions:

Q: What condition is tamsulosin prescribed for?

A: Enlarged prostate (BPH)

Q: What meal-related timing is required for tamsulosin?

A: Take 30 minutes after the same meal daily

#21 Bupropion (WELLBUTRIN)

byoo-PROH-pee-on (WELL-byoo-trin)
Common Uses: Depression, smoking cessation, ADHD (off-label)
Mascot: "Boop ropin' Well booty"

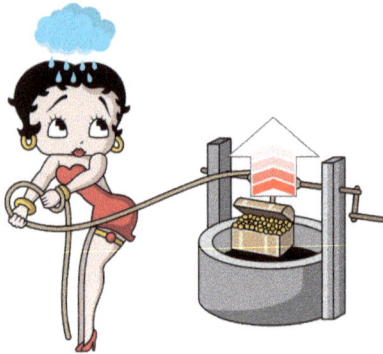

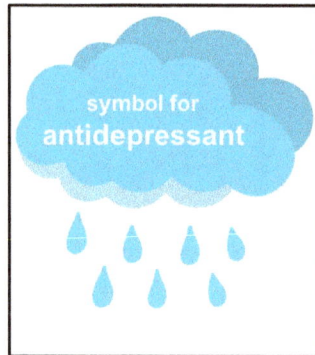

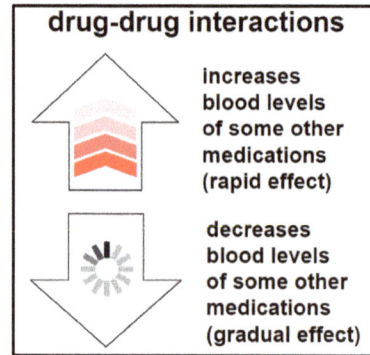

symbol for **antidepressant**

drug-drug interactions

increases blood levels of some other medications (rapid effect)

decreases blood levels of some other medications (gradual effect)

Alternate Mnemonics:
- ❖ "Bu-propels energy and motivation"
- ❖ "Bu-Pro = Boosts Productivity"

Drug Class: Antidepressant: NDRI (Norepinephrine-Dopamine Reuptake Inhibitor)
Similar Drugs: Atomoxetine (#213) – ADHD medication with similar mechanism; Bupropion/Dextromethorphan combo (Auvelity) for depression
Comparisons: No serotonin effects, no sexual dysfunction, more energizing than serotonin antidepressants
Controlled Substance: ☑ Not controlled – although may cause amphetamine-like euphoria at very high dose
High-Alert Risk: ⚠ Seizure risk at high doses or with eating disorders; ⚠ Drug-drug interactions
Major Side Effects: Insomnia, dry mouth, anxiety (uncommon)
Look-Alike/Sound-Alike: Buspirone
Narrow Therapeutic Index: No
Precautions: Not for patients with seizure disorders or eating disorders
Routes: Oral
Formulations: IR = once daily; SR = twice daily; XL = once daily in morning (most used)
Easily Replaceable? No – atomoxetine has similar mechanism but does not work for depression
Also: Increases norepinephrine and dopamine like stimulants, but not classified as one

Sample Test Questions:
Q: What class of antidepressant is bupropion?
A: Norepinephrine-Dopamine Reuptake Inhibitor (NDRI)
Q: Does bupropion usually cause sexual side effects like the SSRIs?
A: No – it typically does not affect sexual function because it has no serotonin effects

#22 Fluoxetine (PROZAC)

FLOO-ox-uh-teen (PRO-zack)

Common Uses: Depression, OCD, anxiety, bulimia, premenstrual dysphoric disorder (PMDD)

Mascot: "Prolonged sack of the Flustered ox"

➤ bull ~ ox → antidepressant of choice for "bull"-imia nervosa

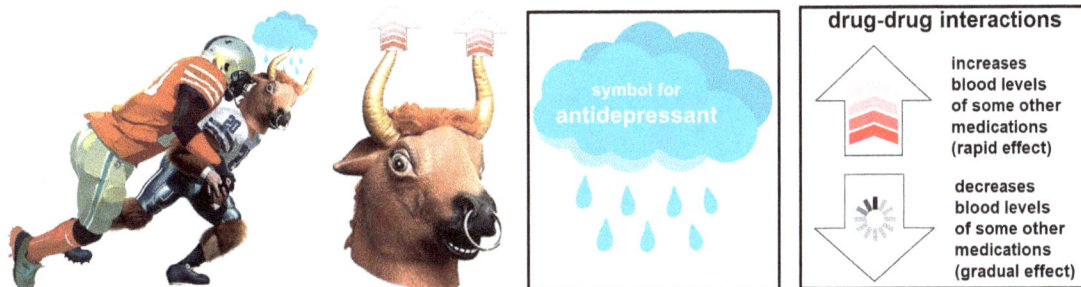

Alternate Mnemonics:

❖ "Fluoxetine floats serotonin levels"

❖ "Prozac's prolonged half-life" = fewer missed-dose effects

Drug Class: Antidepressant: SSRI (Selective Serotonin Reuptake Inhibitor)

Similar SSRIs: Sertraline (#11), Escitalopram (#15), Citalopram (#40), Paroxetine (#92)

Comparisons: Fewer withdrawal symptoms because it has the longest half-life of all SSRIs

Controlled Substance: ✅ Not controlled

High-Alert Risk: ⚠ Drug-drug interactions – for instance it quadruples metoprolol levels

➤ Warning of suicidal thoughts in patients under age 25 – applicable to all antidepressants

➤ Serotonin toxicity – dangerous if combined with a monoamine oxidase inhibitor (MAOI) – phenelzine, tranylcypromine, isocarboxazid, selegiline, linezolid, or methylene blue

Major Side Effects: Insomnia, nausea, sexual dysfunction, anxiety (early)

Look-Alike/Sound-Alike: Fluvoxamine (SSRI approved only for obsessive-compulsive disorder)

Narrow Therapeutic Index: ✅ No – it has a wide therapeutic index

Precautions: Taper is less important due to long half-life – it "tapers itself" down over weeks

Routes: Oral

Easily Replaceable? Partially – SSRIs are similar, but psychiatric medications often require trial and error

Sample Test Questions:

Q: What makes fluoxetine different from other SSRIs?

A: It has the longest half-life

Q: What advantages does fluoxetine have over other SSRIs?

A: Fewer withdrawal symptoms when stopping it or missing a dose (due to long half-life)

Q: What disadvantage does fluoxetine have compared to sertraline and escitalopram?

A: More drug-drug interactions

#23 Hydrocodone/Acetaminophen (VICODIN, NORCO)

hye-DROE-koe-dohn / uh-SEE-tuh-MIN-uh-fen (VY-ko-din)

Common Uses: Moderate to severe pain

Mascot: "Viking Hydrant code"

➤ Opioid mascots have constricted pupils – opioids constrict pupils

➤ See #114 for Acetaminophen mascot info

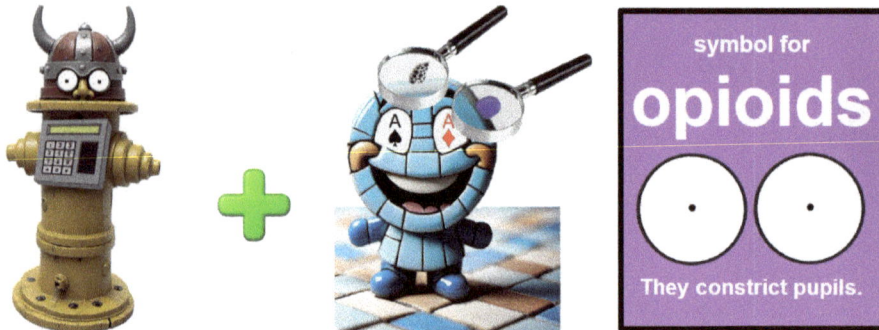

symbol for
opioids

They constrict pupils.

Trade Names: VICODIN, NORCO, LORTAB

Alternate Mnemonics:

❖ "Vicodin: victory over pain, a vice over time"

❖ "Although a narcotic, it's Norco (not Narco)"

❖ "The Vice Squad seized my Vicodin"

Drug Class: Pain reliever: Opioid analgesic + non-opioid (APAP)

Similar Drugs: Oxycodone (#60), Tramadol (#55), Acetaminophen + Codeine (#166)

Comparisons: Weaker than oxycodone; stronger than tramadol

Controlled Substance: ⚠ ⚠ ⚠ C-II – highly addictive

➤ C-II controlled substances (opioids, stimulants) are strictly regulated

High-Alert Risk: ⚠ ⚠ ⚠ ⚠ Among highest-risk meds for overdose and misuse

➤ Contains acetaminophen – liver toxicity risk if taken over max daily dose (4,000 mg)

Major Side Effects: Sedation, constipation, nausea, respiratory depression, addiction

Look-Alike/Sound-Alike: Oxycodone, hydromorphone

Narrow Therapeutic Index: ⚠ Yes – respiratory depression

Precautions: Avoid alcohol and other sedatives. Watch for signs of dependence or misuse.

Routes: Oral

Easily Replaceable? Partially – other opioids may substitute, but dosing and potency vary

Also: The generic name may be displayed as hydrocodone/APAP – APAP is acetaminophen

Sample Test Questions:

Q: What serious liver-related risk comes from this combination?

A: Acetaminophen-induced liver toxicity

#24 Furosemide (LASIX)

fyoor-OH-seh-mide (LAY-six)

Common Uses: Diuretic ("water pill") for edema, heart failure, high blood pressure

Mascot: "Furries see my Laces"

➤ Roller coaster loop → loop diuretic (acting on kidneys at the loop of Henle)

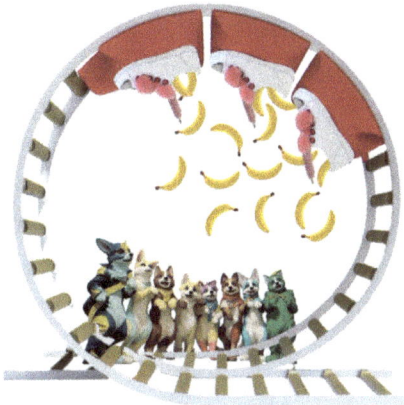

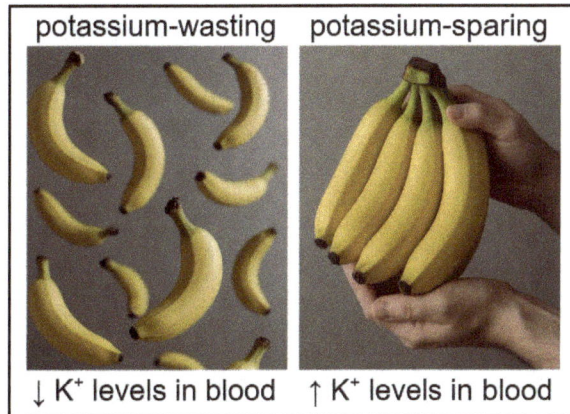

potassium-wasting	potassium-sparing
↓ K^+ levels in blood	↑ K^+ levels in blood

Alternate Mnemonics:

❖ "Furiously removes fluid"

❖ "Lasix = lasts six hours"

❖ "Furosemide floods out potassium"

❖ "Lasix lets go of liquid at the Loop"

Drug Class: Diuretic: Loop diuretic

Similar Drugs: Torsemide (#184), Bumetanide (not top 300), Hydrochlorothiazide (#12)

Comparisons: Stronger and faster than thiazides; causes more potassium loss

High-Alert Risk: ⚠️ ⚠️ Electrolyte depletion (low potassium, low sodium) can lead to cardiac arrhythmias

Major Side Effects: Low potassium, low sodium, dehydration, lightheadedness

Look-Alike/Sound-Alike: Lanoxin, Laxis (non-U.S. brand)

Narrow Therapeutic Index: No

Precautions:

➤ Check potassium levels and kidney function

➤ Can cause hearing loss if given too fast IV

Routes: Oral, IV

Easily Replaceable? Yes – other loop diuretics exist but differ in potency

Sample Test Questions:

Q: What organ function must be monitored with furosemide?

A: Kidney function

Q: Why must IV furosemide be given slowly?

A: Risk of hearing loss (ototoxicity)

#25 Fluticasone (FLONASE nasal, FLOVENT inhaled)

floo-TIK-uh-sone (FLOW-naze, FLOW-vent)
Common Uses: Inhaler for asthma, Nasal spray for allergic rhinitis (runny nose)
Mascot: "Flo's ventilated Flute case"

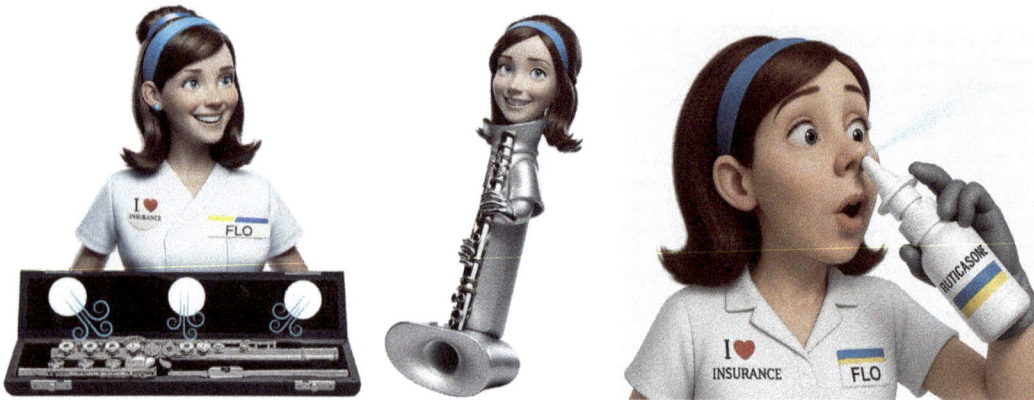

Alternate Mnemonics:

❖ "Flonase flows nasally"

❖ "Flovent ventilates the lungs"

❖ "Fluticasone = fewer sneezes (FLONASE), fewer wheezes (FLOVENT)"

Drug Class: Respiratory anti-inflammatory: Corticosteroid (intranasal, inhaled)
Similar Drugs: Budesonide (#177), Triamcinolone (#102), Mometasone
High-Alert Risk: ✅ Not high alert
Major Side Effects: Nosebleeds, throat irritation
Look-Alike/Sound-Alike: Flunisolide
Narrow Therapeutic Index: No
Precautions: Rinse mouth after inhaled use to prevent thrush (yeast infection of mouth or throat)
Routes: Intranasal, Inhaled
Easily Replaceable? Yes – other nasal and inhaled steroids are comparable
Also: Available OTC in nasal form (FLONASE) but still widely prescribed; Maximum effect may take several days

Sample Test Questions:
Q: What class of medication is fluticasone?
A: Corticosteroid (anti-inflammatory)
Q: How long does it take for fluticasone to reach full effect?
A: Several days
Q: What must patients do after using inhaled fluticasone?
A: Rinse mouth to reduce risk of oral thrush
Q: What form of fluticasone is available over-the-counter (OTC)?
A: Nasal

#26 Amoxicillin (AMOXIL)

uh-MOX-uh-sill-in (uh-MOX-il)
Common Uses: Ear infections, strep throat, sinus infections, urinary tract infections (UTIs)
Mascot: "A Moxy ceiling"

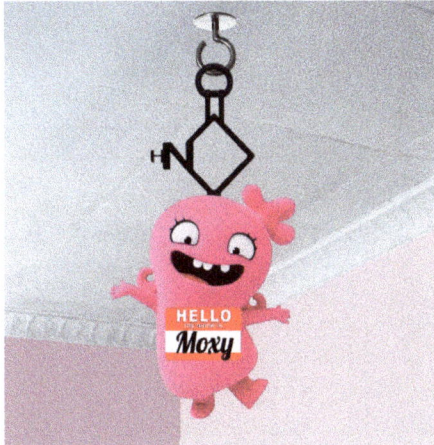

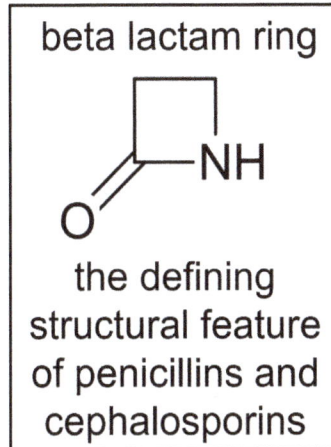

beta lactam ring

the defining structural feature of penicillins and cephalosporins

Alternate Mnemonics:
- ❖ "Ammo against many bugs"
- ❖ "Amoxicillin = all-purpose penicillin"

Drug Class: Antibiotic: Penicillin family (aminopenicillin)
Similar Drugs: Amoxicillin-Clavulanate (#96), Cephalexin (#101)
Comparisons: Greater spectrum of antimicrobial activity compared to penicillin
High-Alert Risk: ✅ Not high alert
Major Side Effects: Rash, diarrhea, allergic reaction
Look-Alike/Sound-Alike: Ampicillin, amiodarone
Narrow Therapeutic Index: ✅ No – it has a wide therapeutic index
Precautions:
- ➤ Not for patients with penicillin allergies
- ➤ Finish full course even if symptoms resolve early – applicable to all antibiotics

Routes: Oral
Easily Replaceable? Yes – cephalosporins often used if mild penicillin allergy

Sample Test Questions:
Q: Are patients with allergy to penicillin likely to have an allergic reaction with amoxicillin?
A: Yes, very likely
Q: Should patients stop amoxicillin when they feel better?
A: No – complete full course – applicable to all antibiotics
Q: Why is amoxicillin often prescribed as amoxicillin/clavulanate combo (Augmentin)?
A. Clavulanate blocks bacterial enzymes that would destroy amoxicillin

#27 Apixaban (ELIQUIS)

uh-PIX-uh-ban (EL-ih-kwiss)

Common Uses: Anticoagulant ("blood thinner") for prevention of stroke in atrial fibrillation (A-fib), Treatment and prevention of deep vein thrombosis (DVT) and pulmonary embolism (PE)

Mascot: "Eloquent pixie ban"

➤ Xaban mascots wear a BANdana and are "banned" (mnemonically, not literally)

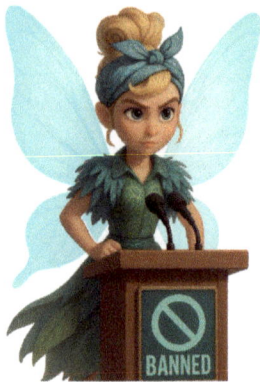

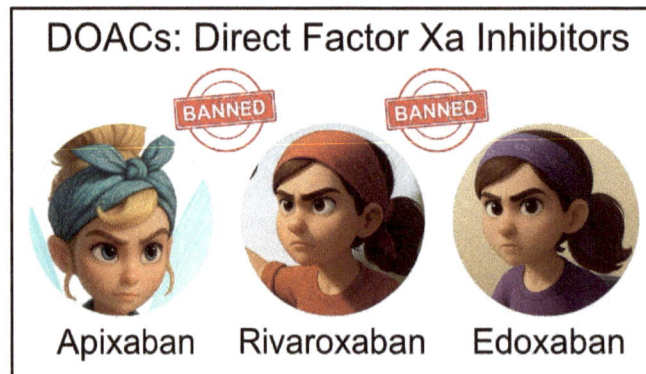

DOACs: Direct Factor Xa Inhibitors

Apixaban   Rivaroxaban   Edoxaban

Alternate Mnemonics:

❖ "Apixaban picks off Factor Xa"

❖ *Apixaban* song on YouTube, Spotify, etc

Drug Class: Anticoagulant: Direct Oral Anticoagulant (DOAC): Factor Xa inhibitor

Similar Drugs: Rivaroxaban (#90), Warfarin (#85)

Comparisons: Shorter half-life, no INR monitoring, fewer food interactions than warfarin

➤ INR (International Normalized Ratio) measures how long blood takes to clot

High-Alert Risk: ⚠️ ⚠️ ⚠️ Major bleeding risk

Major Side Effects: Bleeding, anemia, bruising

Look-Alike/Sound-Alike: Eliquis vs. Exalgo

Narrow Therapeutic Index: No

Precautions: Dose adjustment may be needed in kidney/liver disease

Routes: Oral (the O in DOAC)

Easily Replaceable? Partially – others in class exist but not interchangeable without reassessment

Sample Test Questions:

Q: What clotting factor does apixaban inhibit?

A: Factor Xa (Xa is in its name)

Q: What is a serious risk with apixaban use?

A: Bleeding

Q: Does apixaban require INR monitoring like with warfarin?

A: No

#28 Insulin Glargine (LANTUS)

IN-syoo-lin GLAR-jeen (LAN-tuss)

Common Uses: Type 1 and 2 diabetes

Mascot: "Land us on Glars"

➤ Insulin syringe landing on "Planet Glars"

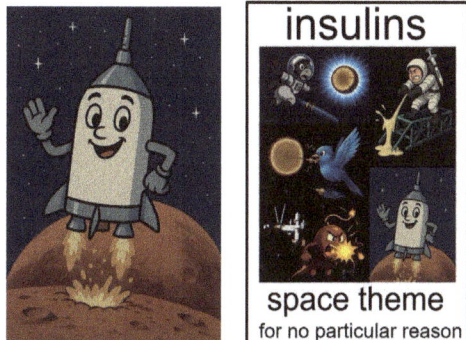

insulins

space theme
for no particular reason

Alternate Mnemonics:

❖ "Glargine glides through the day"

❖ "Lantus = long-lasting like a slow drip"

Drug Class: Long-acting insulin

Similar Drugs: Insulin Detemir (#127), Insulin Degludec (#138)

Comparisons: Lasts ~24 hours with no peak

High-Alert Risk: ⚠ ⚠ ⚠ Risk of severe hypoglycemia (low blood glucose)

Major Side Effects: Low blood sugar, weight gain, injection site reactions

Look-Alike/Sound-Alike: Lente, Levemir

Narrow Therapeutic Index: ⚠ ⚠ ⚠ Yes

Precautions: Monitoring of blood glucose is required

Routes: Subcutaneous injection

Easily Replaceable? No – conversion between long-acting insulins requires careful titration

➤ LANTUS may be replaceable with insulin glargine biosimilars SEMGLEE (without prescriber approval) or BASAGLAR (with provider approval)

Also: Should be administered at the same time each day; Store in fridge before opening; stable at room temp for 28 days

Sample Test Questions:

Q: What type of insulin is glargine?

A: Long-acting

Q: What is a serious risk with insulin glargine?

A: Hypoglycemia – applicable to all insulins

Q: How often is insulin glargine usually given?

A: Once daily

#29 Meloxicam (MOBIC)

meh-LOX-ih-kam (MOH-bick)

Common Uses: Non-steroidal anti-inflammatory drug (NSAID) for pain, osteoarthritis, rheumatoid arthritis

Mascot: "Mel locks a Mobi camel"

➤ "NSAID with long legs" – once daily dosing

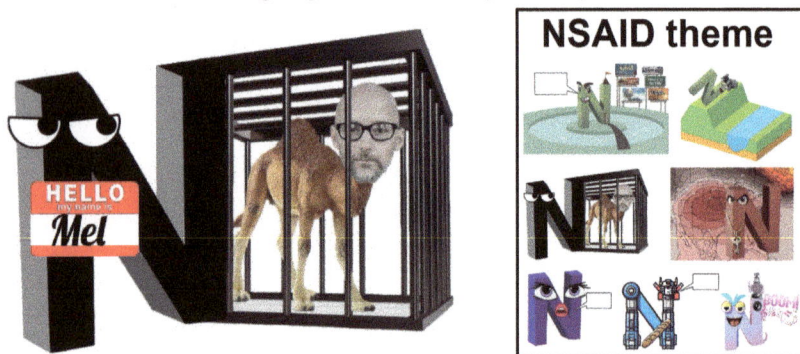

Alternate Mnemonics:

❖ "Meloxicam = mellow out inflammation"

Drug Class: Anti-inflammatory: NSAID (non-steroidal anti-inflammatory drug)

Similar Drugs: Ibuprofen (#33), Naproxen (#89), Celecoxib (#93)

Comparisons: Longer acting → once daily dosing; Compared to ibuprofen/naproxen, meloxicam blocks COX-2 > COX-1 → lower risk of gastric ulcers than ibuprofen/naproxen; Celecoxib is more selective for COX-2 than meloxicam

Controlled Substance: ✅ Not controlled

High-Alert Risk: ⚠️ Risk of GI bleeding, kidney injury

Major Side Effects: GI upset, ulcers, kidney issues, increased BP

Look-Alike/Sound-Alike: Methocarbamol

Narrow Therapeutic Index: No

Precautions:

➤ Avoid in patients with history of ulcers or kidney disease

➤ Use lowest effective dose for shortest time

Routes: Oral

Easily Replaceable? Yes – other NSAIDs available

Sample Test Questions:

Q: What class of medication is meloxicam?

A: NSAID

Q: What organ systems are most at risk with meloxicam use?

A: GI tract and kidneys – applicable to all NSAIDs

Q: What should patients with stomach ulcers avoid?

A: NSAIDs, including meloxicam

#30 Prednisone

PRED-nih-sown (no specific trade name)
Common Uses: Corticosteroid for inflammation, asthma exacerbations, autoimmune diseases
Mascot: "Predator"

➤ Nashville Predators player corticosteroid "moon face"

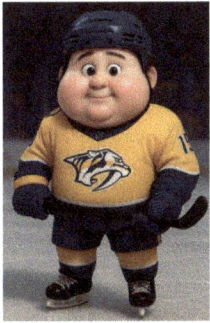

Alternate Mnemonics:

❖ "PREDictable moon face and mood swings"

❖ "Temporary fix with long-term risks"

Drug Class: Anti-inflammatory: Corticosteroid (oral)
Similar Drugs: Methylprednisolone (#153), Dexamethasone (#234), Prednisolone (#136)
Comparisons: Less potent corticosteroid than dexamethasone
High-Alert Risk: ⚠ ⚠ Risks with long-term use; Psychiatric disturbance with short-term use
Major Side Effects: Insomnia, weight gain, high blood sugar, mood changes; psychiatric symptoms in vulnerable patients
Look-Alike/Sound-Alike: Prednisolone
Narrow Therapeutic Index: No
Precautions:

➤ Do not stop suddenly after long-term use

➤ May suppress immune system and adrenal function

Routes: Oral
Easily Replaceable? Yes – other corticosteroids can substitute with dose adjustment
Also: Causes morning energy boost—usually taken early in the day

Sample Test Questions:
Q: What class of drug is prednisone?
A: Corticosteroid
Q: What's a key precaution when stopping prednisone after long use?
A: Taper slowly to avoid adrenal suppression (your body stops making natural steroids)
Q: Name a common mood side effect of prednisone.

#31 Duloxetine (CYMBALTA)

doo-LOX-uh-teen (SIM-ball-tuh)

Common Uses: Depression, anxiety, fibromyalgia, diabetic nerve pain

Mascot: "Dueling Cymbals"

➤ Cymbals may bang the liver → duloxetine can cause liver toxicity (rare)

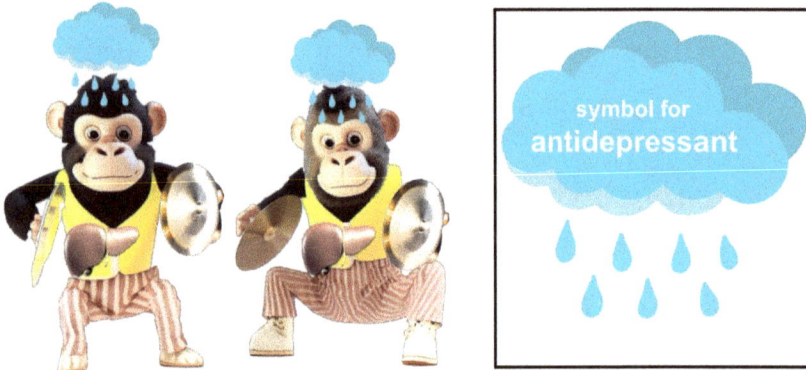

Alternate Mnemonics:

❖ "Dual" mechanism = serotonin + norepinephrine

❖ "Dual" purpose = mood + pain

❖ "Dulo double-duty"

Drug Class: Antidepressant: Serotonin-Norepinephrine Reuptake Inhibitor (SNRI)

Similar SNRIs: Venlafaxine (#44), Desvenlafaxine (#208)

Comparisons: Compared to venlafaxine, duloxetine has more evidence for pain but less evidence for depression

Controlled Substance: ✅ Not controlled

High-Alert Risk: ✅ Not high alert

Major Side Effects: Nausea, dry mouth, sweating, increased BP

Look-Alike/Sound-Alike: Fluoxetine

Narrow Therapeutic Index: No

Precautions:

➤ Warning of suicidal thoughts in patients under age 25 – applicable to all antidepressants

➤ Serotonin toxicity – dangerous if combined with a monoamine oxidase inhibitor (MAOI) – phenelzine, tranylcypromine, isocarboxazid, selegiline, linezolid, or methylene blue

Routes: Oral

Easily Replaceable? Partially – other SNRIs may substitute, but psychiatric meds require trial and error

Sample Test Questions:

Q: Is duloxetine a serotonin reuptake inhibitor?

A: Yes, although it is an SNRI (rather than an SSRI) because it also inhibits reuptake of norepinephrine

#32 Methylphenidate (RITALIN)

METH-ill-FEN-ih-date (RIT-uh-lin)
Common Uses: ADHD, narcolepsy
Mascot: "Write a line on Math final date"

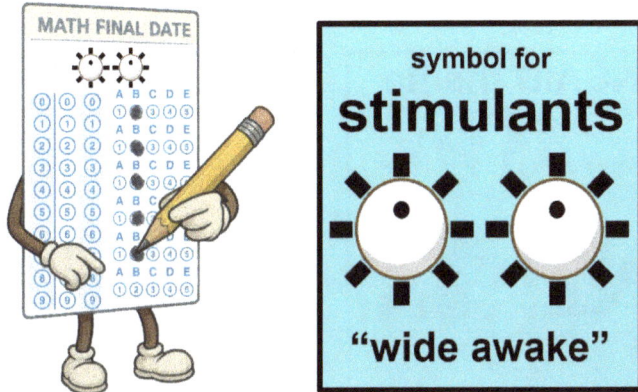

Etymology: Named after the chemist's wife, Rita, who took it to enhance focus while playing tennis
Drug Class: Stimulant: CNS stimulant (dopamine/norepinephrine reuptake inhibitor)
Similar Drugs: Amphetamine salts (#14), Dexmethylphenidate (#109), Lisdexamfetamine (#69)
Comparisons: Shorter-acting than amphetamines; less likely to be abused than amphetamines
Controlled Substance: ⚠ ⚠ ⚠ C-II (Schedule II)

➤ C-II controlled substances (opioids, stimulants) are strictly regulated

High-Alert Risk: ⚠ ⚠ Misuse/abuse risk; affects heart rate and blood pressure
Major Side Effects: Insomnia, decreased appetite, irritability, increased heart rate
Look-Alike/Sound-Alike: Methadone
Narrow Therapeutic Index: No
Precautions:

➤ Do not crush extended-release forms

➤ Monitor growth in children

Formulations: Immediate-release RITALIN is given 2x–3x daily; DAYTRANA is transdermal methylphenidate; CONCERTA is a popular extended-release formulation given once daily
Easily Replaceable? Partially – many formulations differ in onset/duration

Sample Test Questions:
Q: What class of drug is methylphenidate?
A: CNS stimulant
Q: What is a common side effect?
A: Decreased appetite
Q: Name a transdermal version of methylphenidate.
A: DAYTRANA

#33 Ibuprofen (MOTRIN, ADVIL)

eye-byoo-PROH-fen (MOE-trin, AD-vill)
Common Uses: Pain, fever, inflammation
Mascot: "I be pro-Moat in Ad-Ville"

➤ Links generic to both trade names

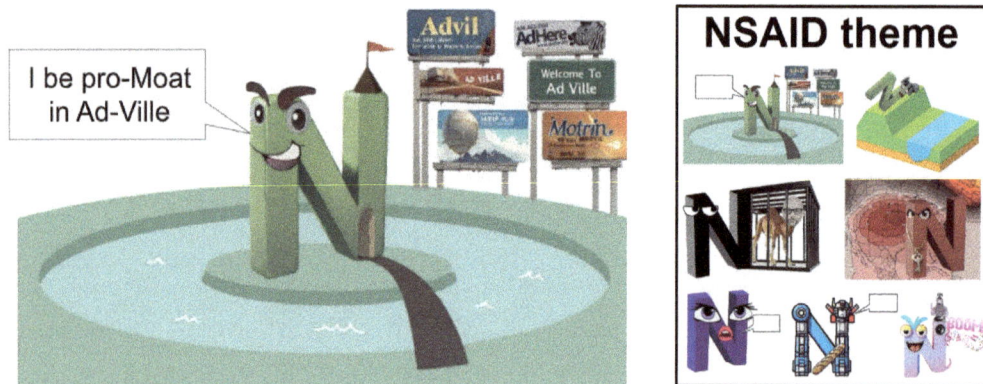

Alternate Mnemonics:

❖ "I take ibuprofen because I-be-broken"

Drug Class: Anti-inflammatory: Non-steroidal anti-inflammatory drug (NSAID)
Similar Drugs: Naproxen (#89), Meloxicam (#29), Diclofenac (#51)
Comparisons: Shorter duration than naproxen; widely available OTC
Controlled Substance: ✅ Not controlled
High-Alert Risk: ⚠ GI bleeding, kidney injury
Major Side Effects: Upset stomach, ulcers, kidney strain, increased blood pressure
Narrow Therapeutic Index: No
Precautions: Take with food to reduce GI risk; Avoid with chronic kidney disease
Routes: Oral, IV
Easily Replaceable? Yes – many NSAIDs available
Also: Available OTC in lower strengths; Prescription only at higher strengths

Sample Test Questions:
Q: What class is ibuprofen in?
A: NSAID
Q: What should patients do to reduce stomach side effects?
A: Take with food
Q: What organ is at risk with long-term NSAID use?
A: Kidneys
Q: What is a gastrointestinal risk of ibuprofen?
A: Stomach ulcers

#34 Carvedilol (COREG)

KAR-veh-dih-lol (KOR-eg)

Common Uses: High blood pressure, after heart attack, heart failure

Mascot: "Corey the Carver"

➤ Beta blockers end in -olol and their mascots wear an "LOL" hat

➤ The polka dots on pink pattern mean it's an alpha-1 blocker – orthostatic hypotension (low blood pressure when standing up) and syncope (fainting) is possible – "hit the floor"

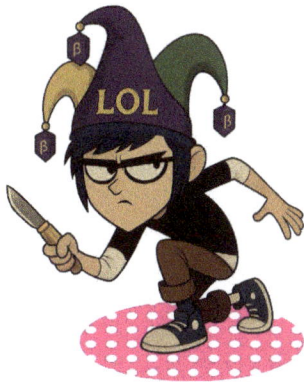

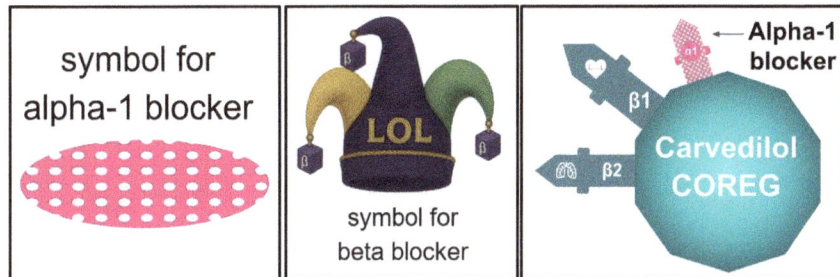

symbol for alpha-1 blocker

symbol for beta blocker

Carvedilol COREG

Alpha-1 blocker

Alternate Mnemonics:

❖ "Coreg = core regulator"

Drug Class: Blood pressure & heart failure: Beta blocker (nonselective) + alpha-1 blocker

Similar Drugs: Metoprolol (#6), Atenolol (#63), Propranolol (#77) – block beta receptors only

Comparisons: In addition to beta blockade, carvedilol reduces peripheral resistance via alpha-1 blockade

High-Alert Risk: ✅ Not high alert

Major Side Effects: Dizziness, fatigue, low heart rate, low blood pressure

Narrow Therapeutic Index: No

Precautions: Monitor heart rate and blood pressure; take with food to reduce orthostatic hypotension (low blood pressure when standing)

Routes: Oral

Easily Replaceable? Partially – other beta blockers available, but few have alpha-blocking effect

➤ Refer to #6 Metoprolol for β blocker comparisons

Sample Test Questions:

Q: What makes carvedilol different from other beta blockers?

A: It also blocks alpha-1 receptors

Q: Why should carvedilol be taken with food?

A: To reduce risk of dizziness (lightheadedness)

#35 Potassium Chloride (K-TAB, KLOR-CON)

puh-TASS-ee-um KLOR-ide (KAY-tab, KLOR-kon)

Common Uses: Hypokalemia (low potassium), diuretic-induced potassium (K+) loss

Mascot: Bananas are known for containing potassium

➤ Celery has an unusually high ~ 3:1 chloride to sodium ratio and "C.L." is a CeLery sound-alike.

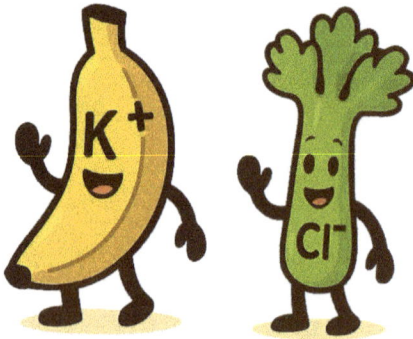

Drug Class: Electrolyte supplement

Similar Drugs: Magnesium salts (#207), Sodium salts (#216)

Comparisons: Commonly used to replace potassium lost by diuretics like furosemide

High-Alert Risk: ⚠️ ⚠️ Risk of severe heart issues if dosing errors occur

Major Side Effects: Nausea, abdominal pain, hyperkalemia (too much K+)

Look-Alike/Sound-Alike: Sodium chloride

Narrow Therapeutic Index: ⚠️ Yes – Too much K+ can cause fatal cardiac arrhythmias

Precautions:

➤ Take with food and full glass of water

➤ Never crush or chew extended-release forms

➤ IV potassium must be diluted; rapid infusion can stop the heart

Routes: Oral, IV

Easily Replaceable? Yes – different salt forms available (e.g., liquid, effervescent)

Also: Often added to Furosemide (#24) or Hydrochlorothiazide (#12), which lower potassium

Sample Test Questions:

Q: What condition is potassium chloride used to treat?

A: Low potassium (hypokalemia)

Q: Why must KCl tablets not be crushed?

A: They are highly concentrated and can cause GI irritation or overdose

Q: What organ is especially sensitive to potassium levels?

A: The heart

#36 Aspirin (ECOTRIN, BAYER), also known as Acetylsalicylic acid (ASA)

ASS-puh-rin (EE-koe-trin, BAY-er, uh-SEE-til-SAL-ih-sill-ik ASS-id)
Common Uses: Heart attack/stroke prevention, pain, inflammation, fever
Mascot:

- ❖ Ecotrin: "Aspirin' Echo trainer"
- ❖ Bayer: "Asa, the Aspirin' Bear"
- ❖ Asa for A.S.A. = Acetylsalicylic acid

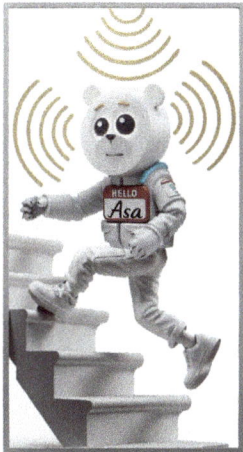

Drug Class: Antiplatelet + NSAID
Similar Drugs: Clopidogrel (#47), Naproxen (#89), Ibuprofen (#33)
Comparisons: Only NSAID used at low doses for heart protection
High-Alert Risk: ⚠️ ⚠️ Risk of gastrointestinal (GI) bleed and Reye's syndrome in children
Major Side Effects: GI upset, bleeding, tinnitus at high doses
Narrow Therapeutic Index: No
Precautions:

- ➤ Avoid in children with viral illness (Reye's syndrome)
- ➤ Can worsen asthma or ulcers

Routes: Oral, rectal
Easily Replaceable? Partially – other antiplatelets exist, but not exact equivalent
Also: Enteric-coated forms reduce GI irritation; Available over-the-counter (OTC)

Sample Test Questions:
Q: What organ-related syndrome can aspirin trigger in children?
A: Reye's syndrome
Q: What dose of aspirin is typically used for heart protection?
A: 81 mg daily (low dose)
Q: What is a major risk of long-term aspirin use?
A: Stomach bleeding

#37 Pravastatin (PRAVACHOL)

PRA-va-stat-in (PRAV-uh-kol)
Common Uses: High cholesterol
Mascot: "Prayin' Prairie statin"

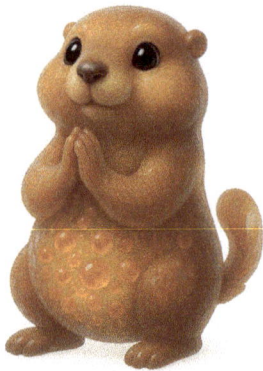

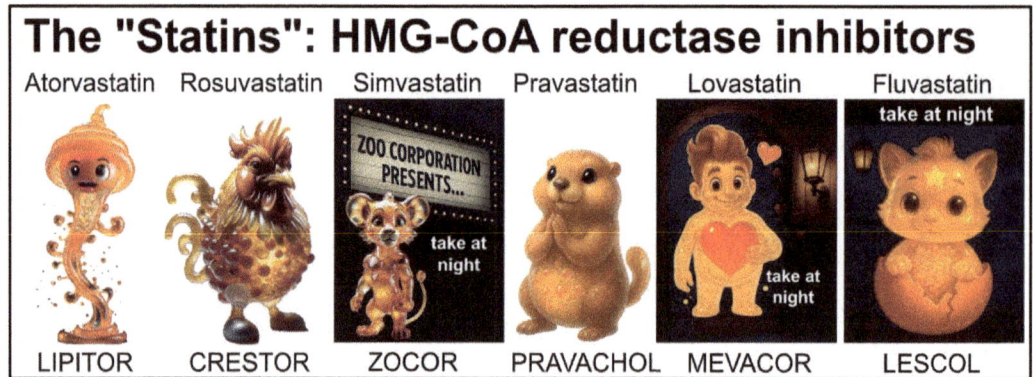

The "Statins": HMG-CoA reductase inhibitors

Atorvastatin — LIPITOR
Rosuvastatin — CRESTOR
Simvastatin — ZOCOR (take at night)
Pravastatin — PRAVACHOL
Lovastatin — MEVACOR (take at night)
Fluvastatin — LESCOL (take at night)

Alternate Mnemonics:

❖ "Pravastatin = proud heart protector"

Drug Class: Cholesterol-lowering: HMG-CoA reductase inhibitor (Statin)
Similar Drugs: Atorvastatin (#1), Rosuvastatin (#13), Simvastatin (#19), Lovastatin (#111)
Comparisons: Less potent but fewer drug interactions than other statins
High-Alert Risk: ✅ Not high alert
Major Side Effects: Muscle aches, liver enzyme elevations
Look-Alike/Sound-Alike: Prevacid
Narrow Therapeutic Index: No
Precautions:

➤ Liver tests recommended – applicable to all statins

Routes: Oral
Easily Replaceable? Yes – several statins available
Also: Can be taken once daily at any time, often with or without food

Sample Test Questions:
Q: What class of drug is pravastatin?
A: Statin
Q: Does pravastatin have a lot of drug interactions?
A: No – fewer than other statins
Q: What lab should be monitored while on pravastatin?
A: Liver enzymes – applicable to all statins

#38 Ergocalciferol (VITAMIN D2)

er-goe-KAL-sih-fer-ol
Common Uses: Vitamin D deficiency
Mascot: "2 Ergonomic D's"

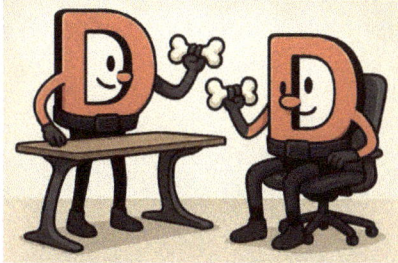

Alternate Mnemonics:

❖ "Ergocalciferol = early treatment of low vitamin D – often started as D2, later switched to D3"

❖ "Ergo" for "erroneous choice" – D3 is usually preferred when available

Drug Class: Vitamin: Vitamin D analog
Similar Drugs: Cholecalciferol (#62), Calcitriol (#254)
Comparisons: Less potent and shorter acting than D3 (cholecalciferol)

➤ D2 is typically given once weekly at a massive dose of 50,000 international units (IU)

➤ D3 is typically given daily at ~ 2,000 IU

High-Alert Risk: ✅ Not high alert
Major Side Effects: Generally none, although may cause high calcium at excessive doses
Look-Alike/Sound-Alike: Calciferol, Calcitriol
Narrow Therapeutic Index: No
Routes: Oral
Easily Replaceable? Yes – cholecalciferol (Vitamin D3)

➤ D3 (cholecalciferol) raises and maintains vitamin D levels better than D2 (ergocalciferol).

Sample Test Questions:
Q: What is another name for ergocalciferol?
A: Vitamin D2
Q: What is a common dosing frequency for ergocalciferol?
A: Once weekly
Q: What should be monitored in high-dose vitamin D therapy?
A: Calcium levels
Q: Which form of vitamin D is more potent and longer-lasting?
A: Cholecalciferol (D3)

#39 Allopurinol (ZYLOPRIM)

al-oh-PYOOR-in-ol (ZYE-lo-prim)

Common Uses: Prevention of gout attacks by reducing uric acid production.

Mascot: "Alli purring"

➤ Purring alligator with a xylophone on his back, referencing Zyloprim trade name

➤ Gout attacks often present as podagra, which is inflammation of the first metatarsophalangeal joint (big toe) due to uric acid crystals

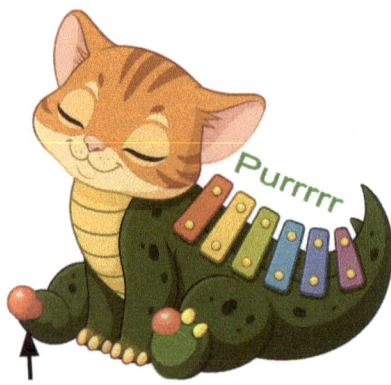

podagra

Alternate Mnemonics:

❖ Zyloprim → "XO-prim" for its mechanism: xanthine oxidase (XO) inhibitor

❖ "Allopurinol stops all purines from becoming uric acid."

Drug Class: Anti-gout: Xanthine oxidase inhibitor

Similar Drugs: Colchicine (#197), Febuxostat (not top 300)

Comparisons: Allopurinol prevents flares; not effective during acute gout attacks like colchicine

High-Alert Risk: ⚠ Rare severe rash (Stevens-Johnson Syndrome)

Major Side Effects: Rash, GI upset, liver enzyme elevations

Look-Alike/Sound-Alike: Alprazolam

Narrow Therapeutic Index: No

Precautions: Starting during an acute gout attack may worsen or prolong the flare

Routes: Oral

Easily Replaceable? Partially – febuxostat is alternative XO inhibitor, but not identical

Also: May be used in cancer patients to prevent uric acid buildup during chemotherapy

Sample Test Questions:

Q: What is the primary use of allopurinol?

A: Gout prevention

Q: Can allopurinol treat an active gout flare?

A: No – it prevents flares, not treats them

Q: What rare but serious side effect is associated with allopurinol?

A: Stevens-Johnson syndrome

#40 Citalopram (CELEXA)

si-TAL-oh-pram (seh-LEX-uh)
Common Uses: SSRI for depression, anxiety
Mascot: "Shitty Lexus Pram"

➤ The "impure" form of escitalopram (LEXAPRO) – no compelling reason to choose it over escitalopram

➤ 50/50 combo of escitalopram (S-citalopram) and an inactive mirror-image molecule (R-citalopram)

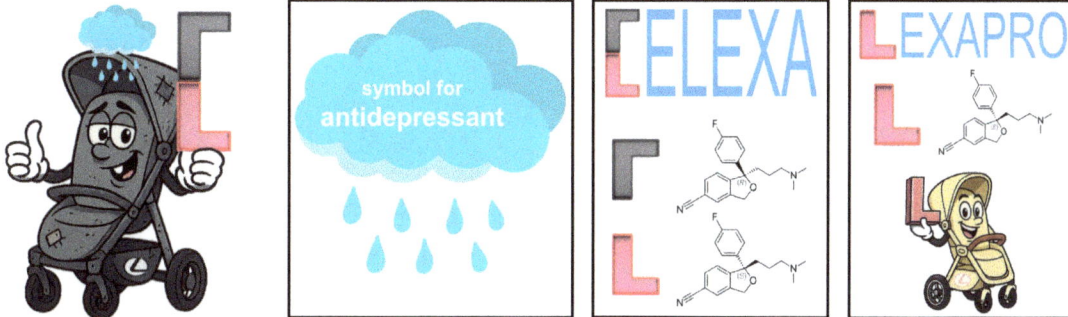

Alternate Mnemonics:

❖ "Citalopram settles serotonin"

❖ "CELEXA = Selects serotonin only"

Drug Class: Antidepressant: Selective Serotonin Reuptake Inhibitor (SSRI)
Similar SSRIs: Escitalopram (#20), Fluoxetine (#10), Sertraline (#5)
Comparisons: Fewer drug interactions than fluoxetine or paroxetine

➤ More QT prolongation (slowed cardiac conduction) at high doses than other SSRIs

◇ Overdose fatality rate ≈ 1 in 2,500, vs. ≈ 1 in 10,000 for escitalopram

✅ Citalopram is generally safe, but escitalopram has a better safety profile

Controlled Substance: ✅ Not controlled

High-Alert Risk: ⚠ Minor risk of QT prolongation (cardiac conduction abnormality); Warning of suicidal thoughts in patients under age 25 – applicable to all antidepressants

➤ Risk of serious serotonin toxicity if combined with a monoamine oxidase inhibitor (MAOI)

Major Side Effects: Nausea, sexual dysfunction
Look-Alike/Sound-Alike: Celecoxib, Escitalopram
Narrow Therapeutic Index: ✅ No – it has a wide therapeutic index
Precautions: Taper slowly to avoid serotonin withdrawal symptoms
Easily Replaceable? Yes —10 mg of escitalopram is equivalent to 20 mg of citalopram—and may be more effective due to its purified, active form. Doctor's order is required for substitution.

Sample Test Questions:
Q: What heart effect can occur with high-dose citalopram?
A: QT prolongation

#41 Alprazolam (XANAX)

al-PRAY-zoe-lam (ZAN-ax)
Common Uses: Anxiety, panic disorder
Mascot: "Lil' Xan, Alp-raised lamb"

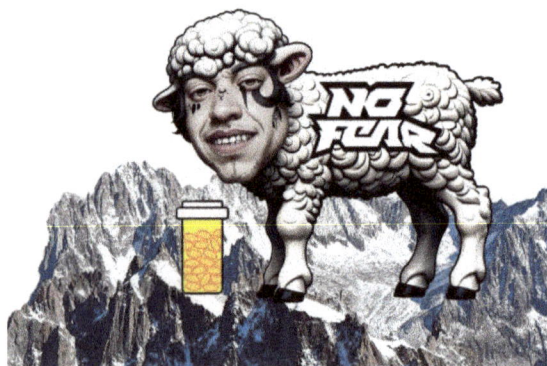

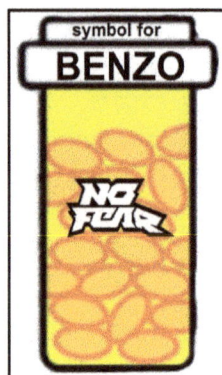

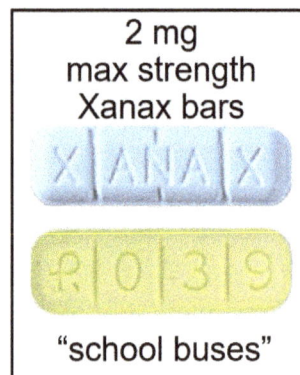

symbol for
BENZO

2 mg
max strength
Xanax bars

"school buses"

Drug Class: Anxiolytic: Benzodiazepine
Similar Drugs: Lorazepam (#81), Diazepam (#169), Clonazepam (#57)
Comparisons: Faster acting than most benzos; more potent for panic; higher abuse potential
Controlled Substance: ⚠ C-IV (Schedule IV)
High-Alert Risk: ⚠ ⚠ ⚠ Risk of respiratory depression, falls, and dependence
Major Side Effects: Drowsiness, dizziness, memory issues, dependence
Look-Alike/Sound-Alike: Lorazepam
Narrow Therapeutic Index: No
Precautions:
> ➤ Avoid with alcohol or opioids – risk of respiratory depression and death
> ➤ Avoid abrupt discontinuation due to potentially dangerous withdrawal with seizures

Routes: Oral
Easily Replaceable? Yes – benzodiazepines are comparable with defined dose conversions
Also: Fast onset makes it more prone to misuse; Benzo withdrawal symptoms resemble alcohol withdrawal

Sample Test Questions:
Q: How is alprazolam different from other benzodiazepines?
A: It is faster-acting, more potent, and more likely to be abused
Q: What's a serious risk when combining alprazolam with opioids?
A: Respiratory depression, ↑ risk of death – applicable to all benzos
Q: What DEA class is alprazolam?
A: C-IV (Schedule IV) – applicable to all benzos

#42 Glipizide (GLUCOTROL)

GLIP-ih-zide (GLOO-koe-troll)
Common Uses: Type 2 diabetes
Mascot: "Clip a side for Glucose control"

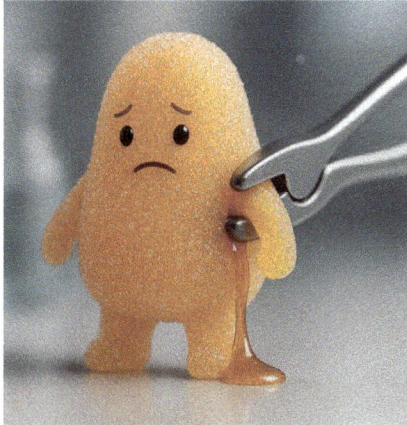

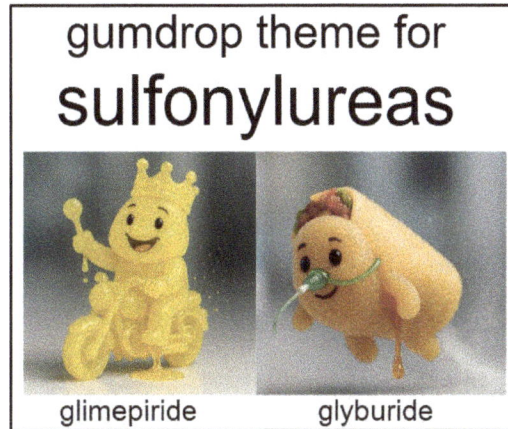

gumdrop theme for
sulfonylureas

glimepiride   glyburide

Alternate Mnemonics:

❖ "Glipizide glides sugar down"

❖ "Glucotrol controls glucose by squeezing insulin out of the pancreas"

❖ *Glipizide* song available on YouTube, Spotify, etc

Drug Class: Antidiabetic: Sulfonylurea

Similar Drugs: Glimepiride (#64), Glyburide (#187)

Comparisons: Shorter-acting than glyburide; less hypoglycemia in elderly

High-Alert Risk: ⚠ ⚠ Risk of hypoglycemia

Major Side Effects: Hypoglycemia, weight gain, nausea

Look-Alike/Sound-Alike: Glimepiride

Narrow Therapeutic Index: No

Precautions:

➤ Eat meals regularly to avoid low blood sugar

Routes: Oral

Easily Replaceable? Yes – other sulfonylureas are comparable

Also: Not effective in patients with severely reduced pancreatic function; Most sulfa-allergic patients can take sulfonylureas, but check if the allergy was severe.

Sample Test Questions:

Q: What class is glipizide?

A: Sulfonylurea

Q: Should patients skip meals when taking glipizide?

A: No – risk of low blood sugar

#43 Cetirizine (ZYRTEC)

seh-TEER-ih-zeen (ZUR-tek)
Common Uses: Allergic rhinitis (runny nose), urticaria (hives)
Mascot: "Sir Tech, the Sitter"

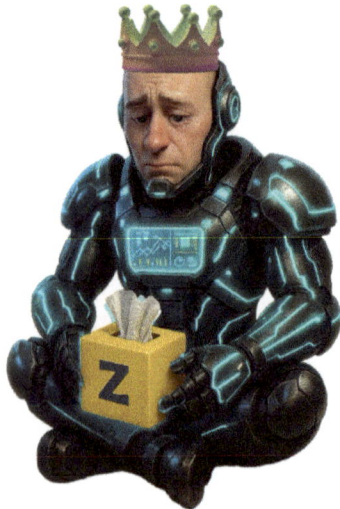

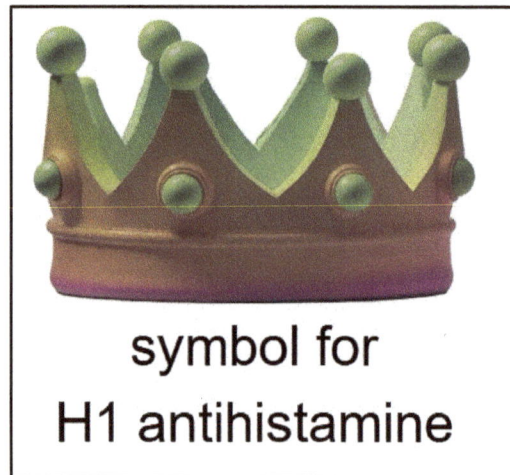

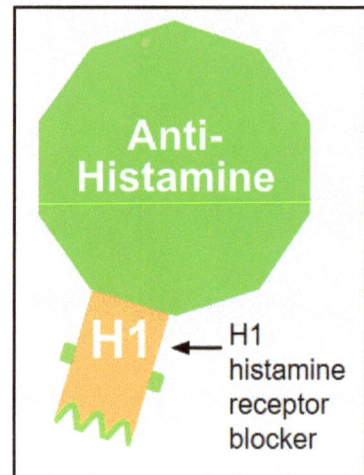

symbol for
H1 antihistamine

Anti-Histamine

H1

← H1 histamine receptor blocker

Alternate Mnemonics:

❖ "ZYRTEC = zero sneezing"

❖ "Cetirizine = see tears gone" (from allergic conjunctivitis)

Drug Class: Antihistamine: 2nd-generation H1 blocker (antihistamine)
Similar Drugs: Loratadine (#72), Fexofenadine (#257), Diphenhydramine (#258)
Comparisons: Less sedating than diphenhydramine; slightly more sedating than loratadine
Controlled Substance: ✅ Not controlled
High-Alert Risk: ✅ Not high alert
Major Side Effects: Drowsiness, dry mouth, fatigue
Look-Alike/Sound-Alike: Sertraline
Narrow Therapeutic Index: ✅ No
Routes: Oral
Easily Replaceable? Yes – other 2nd-gen antihistamines available
Also: Available OTC and widely used for seasonal allergies

Sample Test Questions:
Q: What class is cetirizine?
A: Antihistamine (2nd generation)
Q: Does cetirizine cause drowsiness?
A: Less than diphenhydramine, but possible
Q: What is cetirizine used to treat?
A: Allergies and hives

#44 Venlafaxine (EFFEXOR XR)

VEN-la-fax-een (EF-ex-or)

Common Uses: SNRI for depression, anxiety

Mascot: "Vanilla e-Faxing"

➤ 1980s rapper Vanilla Ice

➤ Blood pressure cuff → Venlafaxine may increase blood pressure

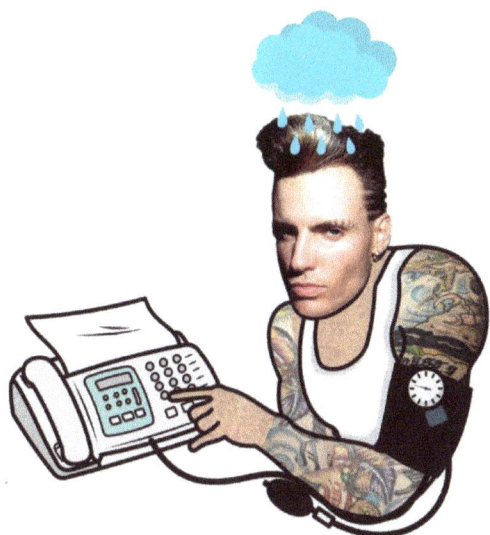

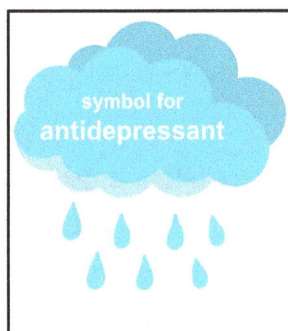

symbol for antidepressant

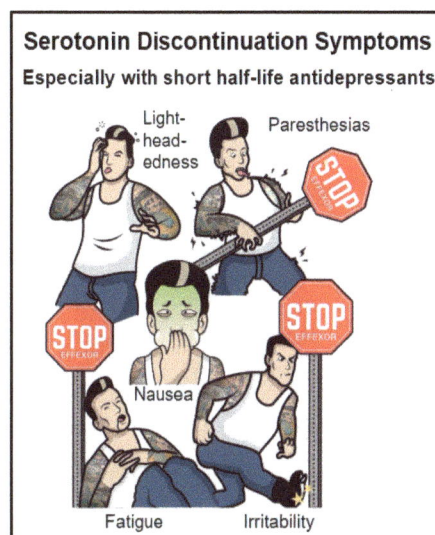

Serotonin Discontinuation Symptoms
Especially with short half-life antidepressants

Light-head-edness · Paresthesias · STOP · Nausea · STOP · Fatigue · Irritability

Alternate Mnemonics:

❖ "EFFEXOR = effects on dual transmitters" – serotonin and norepinephrine

❖ "Effective for depression"

Drug Class: Antidepressant: Serotonin-Norepinephrine Reuptake Inhibitor (SNRI)

Similar Drugs: Duloxetine (#33), Desvenlafaxine (#208)

Comparisons: More serotonergic at low doses, adds norepinephrine reuptake inhibition as dose increases

Controlled Substance: ✅ Not controlled

High-Alert Risk: ✅ Not high alert

Major Side Effects: Nausea, insomnia, increased blood pressure, withdrawal symptoms

Narrow Therapeutic Index: No

Precautions: Do not stop abruptly – withdrawal symptoms can be severe; Monitor blood pressure, especially at higher doses

Routes: Oral

Easily Replaceable? Partially – SNRIs are similar, but psychiatric medications often require trial and error

Also: Extended-release (XR) form preferred for smoother effect and fewer side effects

➤ The original immediate-release (IR) venlafaxine was nicknamed "Side-Effexoer"

Sample Test Questions:

Q: What side effect may be seen with high-dose venlafaxine?

A: High blood pressure

#45 Cyclobenzaprine (FLEXERIL)

SYE-kloe-BEN-zuh-preen (FLEX-er-ill)
Common Uses: Muscle spasms, back pain
Mascot: "Flexible Cycle bending"

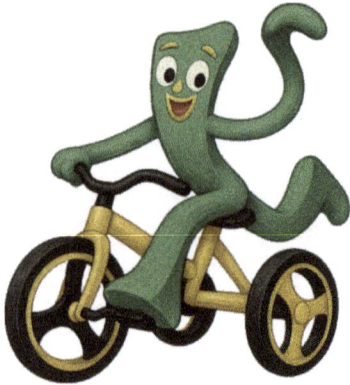

Drug Class: Muscle relaxant: Centrally acting skeletal muscle relaxant
➤ Centrally acting means it works in the brain or spinal cord, not directly on muscles
Similar Drugs: Tizanidine (#94), Baclofen (#104), Methocarbamol (#126)
Comparisons: More sedating than methocarbamol
Controlled Substance: ✅ Not controlled
➤ Among muscle relaxants, the only controlled substance is carisoprodol (Soma)
High-Alert Risk: ⚠️ Drowsiness, fall risk
Major Side Effects: Drowsiness, dry mouth, dizziness
Look-Alike/Sound-Alike: Cyclophosphamide, Cycloserine
Narrow Therapeutic Index: No
Precautions: Avoid alcohol and other CNS depressants
Routes: Oral
Easily Replaceable? Yes – several muscle relaxants available
Also: Not recommended for chronic use; usually for less than 2–3 weeks

Sample Test Questions:
Q: What is cyclobenzaprine used for?
A: Muscle spasms
Q: What's a common side effect of cyclobenzaprine?
A: Drowsiness
Q: What class is cyclobenzaprine in?
A: Muscle relaxants

#46 Hydroxyzine (ATARAX, VISTARIL)

hye-DROX-uh-zeen (VISS-tuh-ril, AT-uh-rax)
Common Uses: Allergies, anxiety, insomnia, nausea
Mascot: "Hydrozoan's Atari" & "Hydrozoan's Vest roll"

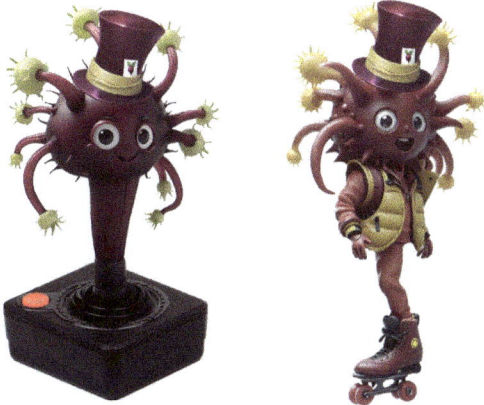

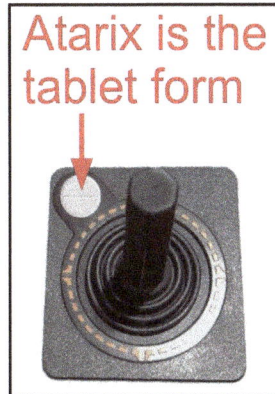

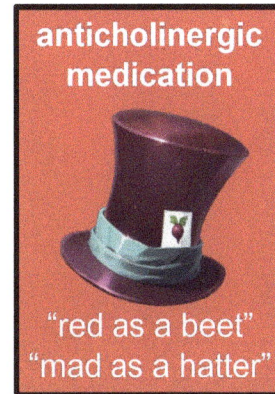

Atarix is the tablet form

anticholinergic medication

"red as a beet"
"mad as a hatter"

Alternate Mnemonics:

❖ "Hydra zips anxiety away"

❖ "Vistaril = very still mind" – used for anxiety and insomnia

❖ "Atarax attacks anxiety"

❖ "H1 = one chill head" (antihistamine)

Drug Class: Antihistamine: H1 receptor antagonist (1st generation)
Similar Drugs: Diphenhydramine, Cetirizine, Loratadine
Comparisons: More sedating than 2nd-gen antihistamines like cetirizine or loratidine
Controlled Substance: ✅ Not controlled
High-Alert Risk: ✅ Not high alert
Major Side Effects: Drowsiness, dry mouth, dizziness, confusion
Look-Alike/Sound-Alike: Hydralazine
Narrow Therapeutic Index: ✅ No – it has a wide therapeutic index
Precautions: Caution in elderly due to anticholinergic effects
Routes: Oral, intramuscular (IM)
Easily Replaceable? Yes – diphenhydramine (Benadryl) is similar
Also: Sometimes used for anxiety instead of benzodiazepines

Sample Test Questions:
Q: What class is hydroxyzine?
A: First-generation antihistamine (H1 blocker)
Q: What side effect is most common?
A: Drowsiness
Q: Is hydroxyzine a controlled substance?
A: No

#47 Clopidogrel (PLAVIX)

klo-PID-oh-grel (PLAV-iks)
Common Uses: Prevent heart attack, stroke, or stent thrombosis
Mascot: "Platelet Clopper grill"

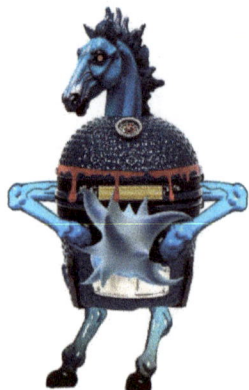

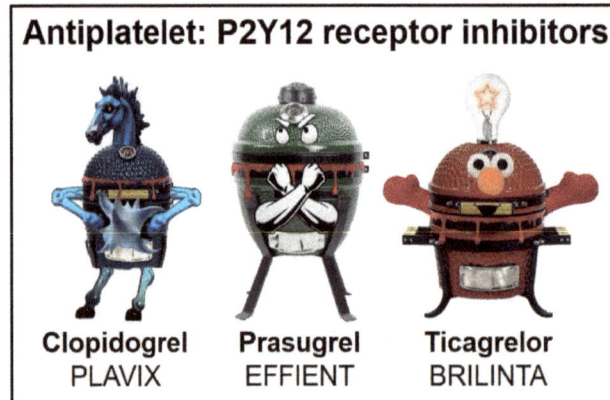

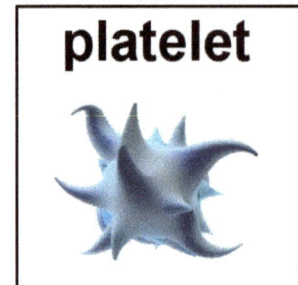

Antiplatelet: P2Y12 receptor inhibitors

Clopidogrel PLAVIX | Prasugrel EFFIENT | Ticagrelor BRILINTA

platelet

Alternate Mnemonics:
- ❖ "Clopid = clot-bid farewell"
- ❖ "Plavix = platelets vanish"
- ❖ "Clop the clots"

Drug Class: Antithrombotic ("blood thinner"): Antiplatelet: P2Y12 receptor inhibitor
➤ P2Y12 receptors are found on platelets

Similar Drugs: Ticagrelor (#203), Prasugrel (>#300)
Comparisons: Safer than ticagrelor in older adults
High-Alert Risk: ⚠️ ⚠️ Risk of serious bleeding, especially around surgery or with other antithrombotics
Major Side Effects: Bruising (minor bleeding under skin), serious bleeding, rash, GI discomfort
Look-Alike/Sound-Alike: Plavix vs. Paxil
Narrow Therapeutic Index: No
Precautions:
➤ Do not discontinue abruptly after a coronary stent (metal tube placed to keep the artery open)
➤ Use caution with NSAIDs (↑ bleeding from platelet effects + GI irritation)
Routes: Oral
Easily Replaceable? Yes – other drugs in this class are comparable

Sample Test Questions:
Q: What is clopidogrel commonly used for?
A: To prevent heart attacks and strokes
Q: What is the major clinical risk associated with clopidogrel?
A: Bleeding

#48 Semaglutide (RYBELSUS, OZEMPIC, WEGOVY)

sem-a-GLOO-tide (ry-BEL-sus, oh-ZEM-pick, WEG-oh-vee)

Common Uses: Type 2 diabetes, weight loss

Mascot: "(Rebel, Olympic, & Wig governor) See my glue tide"

➤ The mascots are wearing glasses to "see" the glue tide

➤ The Rebel says "You ain't injectin' me!" – Rebelsus is taken by mouth, the others subcutaneously

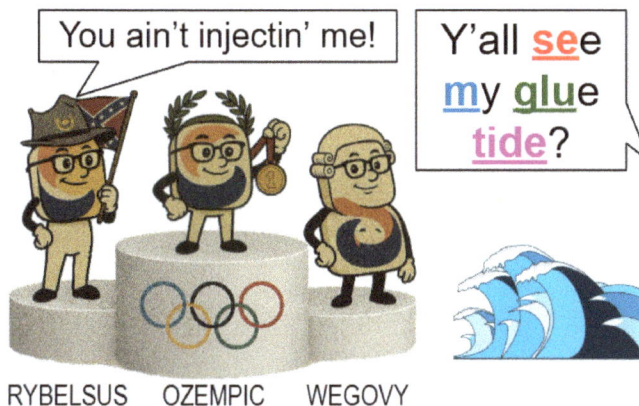

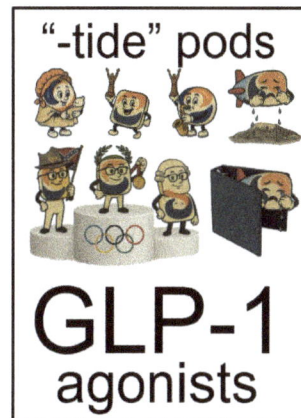

Alternate Mnemonics:

❖ "GLUTide = glucose-lowering tide"

❖ WEGOVY = "weight go away" / "we gon' lose weight with Wegovy" / "weekly Wegovy"

➤ Wegovy is the brand approved for weight loss even without diabetes

❖ GLP-1 = "gut loss power" / "glucose lowering power" / "gotta lose pounds"

Drug Class: Antidiabetic: GLP-1 receptor agonist

Similar Drugs: Liraglutide (#139), Dulaglutide (#74), Tirzepatide (New)

Comparisons: WEGOVY causes less weight loss than tirzepatide (MOUNJARO, ZEPBOUND), but more weight loss than others; All GLP-1 agonists are subcutaneous injections except for RYBELSUS

High-Alert Risk: ⚠ ⚠ Pancreatitis, thyroid tumor risk; Must be held prior to surgery because delayed stomach emptying can lead to aspiration (stomach contents breathed into lungs) under anaesthesia

Major Side Effects: Nausea, vomiting

Narrow Therapeutic Index: No

Precautions: Contraindicated with personal/family history of medullary thyroid cancer; Titrate slowly to reduce GI effects

Routes: Oral (Rybelsus), SubQ (Ozempic, Wegovy)

Easily Replaceable? Yes – other GLP-1 agonists are comparable

Sample Test Questions:

Q: How often is semaglutide injected?

A: Once weekly

Q: What serious side effect may occur with GLP-1 agonists?

A: Pancreatitis

#49 Famotidine (PEPCID)

fa-MOH-ti-deen (PEP-sid)
Common Uses: Acid reducer for gastroesophageal reflux disease (GERD)
Mascot: "Pepsi Family tidings"

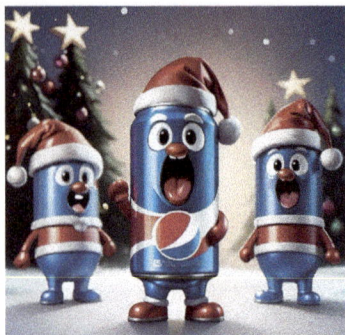

Alternate Mnemonics:

- ❖ "Pepcid = peptic acid reducer"
- ❖ "Fam = family dinner without heartburn"
- ❖ "Famotidine = Acidic fam? Tame it down"

Drug Class: Acid Reducer: H2 histamine receptor antagonist (H2 antihistamine)
Similar Drugs: Nizatidine (>#300), Cimetidine (>#300)
Comparisons: Fewer side effects and drug interactions than cimetidine; Safer but less powerful than proton pump inhibitors (PPIs) like omeprazole or pantoprazole
High-Alert Risk: ✅ Not high alert
Major Side Effects: Headache, constipation, diarrhea, dizziness
Look-Alike/Sound-Alike: Pepcid vs. Prevacid
Narrow Therapeutic Index: ✅ No – it has a wide therapeutic index
Precautions: No major precautions
Routes: Oral, IV
Easily Replaceable? Yes – other H2 blockers are comparable
Also: Available over-the-counter (OTC)

Sample Test Questions:
Q: Is famotidine available over-the-counter?
A: Yes
Q: What condition does it treat?
A: GERD – commonly pronounced "gerd", not "G.E.R.D."
Q: What class is famotidine?
A: H2 blocker (H2 histamine receptor antagonist)
Q: How are H2 blockers different from proton pump inhibitors?
A: H2 blockers are safer but less powerful

#50 Estradiol (ESTRACE)

ess-truh-DYE-ol (ESS-trayss)
Common Uses: Menopausal symptoms or low estrogen levels
Mascot: "Es-trojan horse"

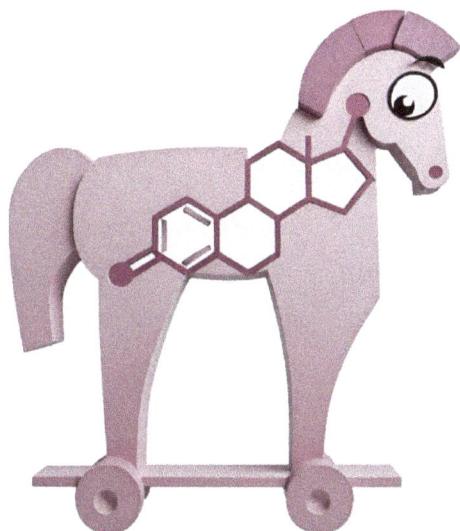

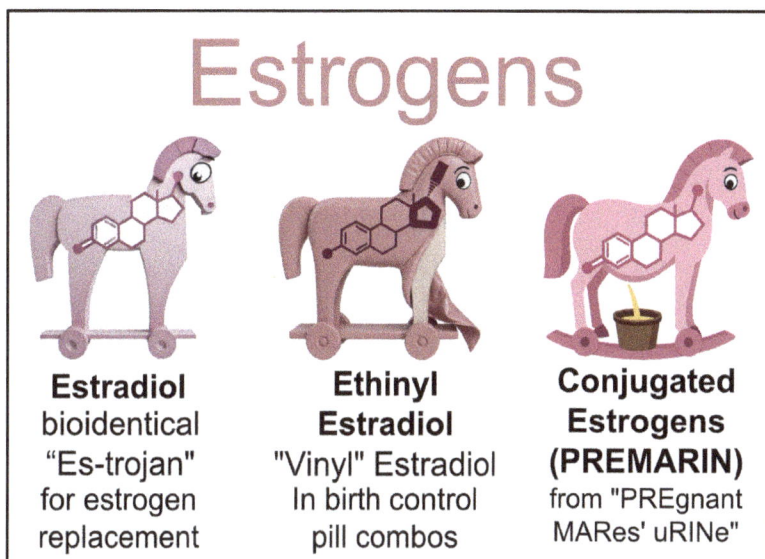

Estrogens

Estradiol
bioidentical
"Es-trojan"
for estrogen
replacement

Ethinyl Estradiol
"Vinyl" Estradiol
In birth control
pill combos

Conjugated Estrogens (PREMARIN)
from "PREgnant MARes' uRINe"

Drug Class: Hormone: Estrogen
Similar Drugs: Ethinyl Estradiol combos (#80, #99, #128, etc.); Conjugated Estrogens (>#300)
Comparisons: Estradiol is identical to natural E2, the most potent *natural* form of estrogen
- ➤ Ethinyl estradiol, found in most birth control pills, is more potent than estradiol
- ➤ Conjugated estrogens (Premarin) are from Pregnant MARes' urINe (hence the name)

Controlled Substance: ☑ Not controlled
High-Alert Risk: ⚠ ⚠ Blood clots, cancer risk
Major Side Effects: Breast tenderness, mood changes, spotting
Look-Alike/Sound-Alike: Estrace vs. Estrogel
Narrow Therapeutic Index: No
Precautions: Use lowest effective dose for shortest duration
Routes: Oral, transdermal, vaginal
Easily Replaceable? No – this drug has unique properties or uses
Also: Transdermal patch has lower risk of blood clots than the pill

Sample Test Questions:
Q: What serious risk is associated with estradiol?
A: Blood clots
Q: Why is the transdermal patch often preferred over the pill?
A: Lower risk of blood clots

#51 Diclofenac (VOLTAREN)

di-KLOE-fen-ak (VOL-tair-en, FLEK-tor, CAM-bee-uh)
Common Uses: Pain, arthritis
Mascot: "Dick Loaf Voltron"

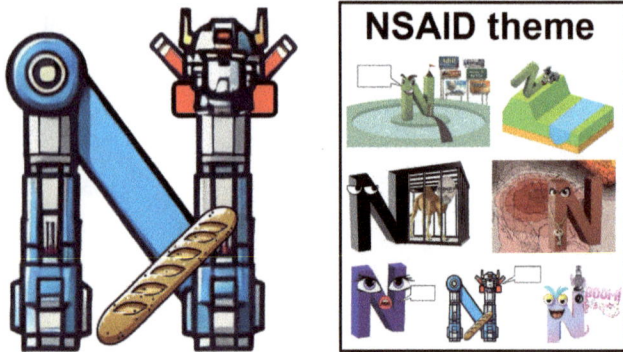

Alternate Mnemonics:

❖ "Diclo dices inflammation"

Drug Class: Anti-inflammatory: NSAID (non-selective COX inhibitor)
Similar Drugs: Meloxicam (#29), Ibuprofen (#33), Naproxen (#89)
Comparisons: More GI and cardiovascular risk than naproxen
Controlled Substance: ✅ Not controlled

High-Alert Risk: ⚠️ ⚠️ Risk of GI bleeding and cardiovascular events
Major Side Effects: GI upset, ulcers, increased blood pressure, kidney impairment
Look-Alike/Sound-Alike: Diphenhydramine
Narrow Therapeutic Index: No
Precautions:

➤ Avoid in patients with recent heart attack or GI bleeding

➤ Take with food to minimize GI irritation

Routes: Oral, topical, IV
Easily Replaceable? Yes – other NSAIDs are comparable
Also: Available as Voltaren gel, patch, and Cambia powder for migraine

Sample Test Questions:
Q: What class is diclofenac?
A: NSAID (non-selective COX inhibitor)
Q: What are major risks of NSAIDs like diclofenac?
A: GI bleeding and cardiovascular events
Q: Is diclofenac a controlled substance?
A: No – NSAIDs are not controlled
Q: What's a topical form of diclofenac?
A: Voltaren gel

#52 Spironolactone (ALDACTONE)

spir-ON-oh-lak-tone (AL-dak-tone)

Common Uses: Diuretic ("water pill") for heart failure, high blood pressure; Also a testosterone blocker used for acne, hirsutism (facial hair in females), gender-affirming treatment in transgender women, polycystic ovary syndrome (PCOS)

Mascot: "Aldosterone redactor's Spiral lactose cone"

➤ Bananas stuck to ice cream → potassium sparing → increases blood K^+ levels

➤ "Aldosterone redactor" → blocks aldosterone's effects on sodium and potassium in kidney

➤ The mascot has pink breasts → spironolactone inhibits testosterone synthesis and can cause breast growth in men

➤ SpironoLACTone – think lactose in ice cream, lactation

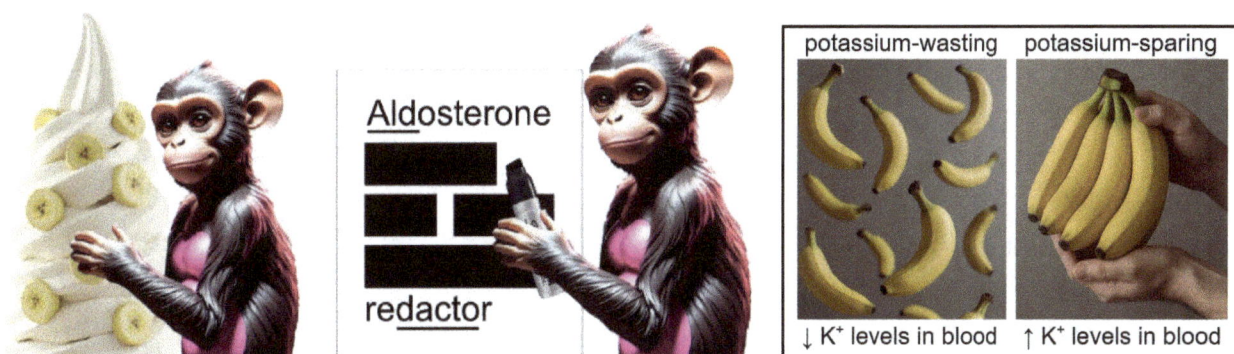

potassium-wasting | potassium-sparing
↓ K^+ levels in blood | ↑ K^+ levels in blood

Drug Class: Diuretic: Potassium-sparing, aldosterone antagonist

Similar Drugs: Eplerenone (>#300)

Comparisons: Less potent diuretic effect than loop or thiazide diuretics

High-Alert Risk: ⚠ Can cause life-threatening hyperkalemia (high K^+) in kidney disease

Major Side Effects: Hyperkalemia, gynecomastia (breast growth), menstrual changes

Look-Alike/Sound-Alike: Aldactazide

Narrow Therapeutic Index: No

Precautions: Monitor potassium and kidney function closely; Avoid potassium supplements

Routes: Oral

Easily Replaceable? No – this drug has unique properties or uses

Sample Test Questions:

Q: What electrolyte abnormality can spironolactone cause?

A: Hyperkalemia (high potassium)

Q: What hormone does spironolactone antagonize?

A: Aldosterone

Q: What conditions is spironolactone commonly used for, related to its anti-testosterone effects?

A: Acne and polycystic ovary syndrome (PCOS)

#53 Hydrochlorothiazide + Lisinopril (ZESTORETIC)

hye-droe-klor-oh-THYE-a-zide; lyse-IN-oh-pril

Common Uses: Hypertension

Mascot: "Micro Hydrant, tie-dyed" (#12) + "Licensed Zest drill" (#3)

➤ Hydrochlorothiazide (HCTZ) lowers potassium (K^+) by causing it to be lost in the urine, while lisinopril increases K^+ by helping the body keep it → K^+ effects may balance out, leading to more stable potassium levels

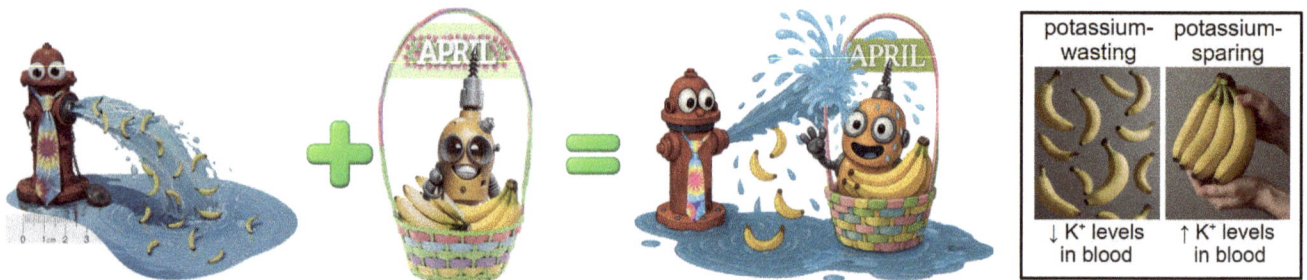

potassium-wasting	potassium-sparing
↓ K^+ levels in blood	↑ K^+ levels in blood

Alternate Mnemonics:

❖ "Hydro-Lisin = hydration + ACE-in"

Drug Class: Antihypertensive: ACE inhibitor + thiazide diuretic

Similar Drugs: Losartan/HCTZ (#75)

Comparisons: Similar combo effects; cough more likely than with losartan/HCTZ

High-Alert Risk: ⚠ Hypotension (low blood pressure), hyperkalemia (high potassium, lisinopril) or angioedema (serious swelling, lisinopril)

Major Side Effects: Cough (lisinopril), dizziness, low sodium (HCTZ)

Look-Alike/Sound-Alike: Lisinopril vs. Losartan

Narrow Therapeutic Index: No

Precautions: Avoid in pregnancy – risk of birth defects; Monitor electrolytes and renal function

Routes: Oral

Easily Replaceable? Yes – other ACE inhibitor or angiotensin II receptor blocker (ARB) + HCTZ combos are comparable

Sample Test Questions:

Q: What class is lisinopril?

A: ACE inhibitor

Q: What serious side effect is linked to ACE inhibitors?

A: Angioedema

Q: Should this combo be used in pregnancy?

A: No

Q: What does hydrochlorothiazide do?

A: Increases sodium and water excretion

#54 Buspirone (BUSPAR)

BYOO-spi-rone (BYOO-spar)
Common Uses: Generalized anxiety disorder (GAD)
Mascot: "Bus Spear"

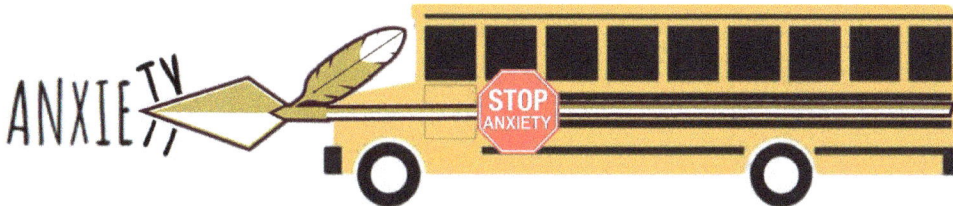

Alternate Mnemonics:

❖ "Buspirone boosts calm, not sedation"

❖ "Takes time to work, no buzz" – slower to work than benzodiazepines (benzos), not abusable

❖ "Buspar is benign" – not the strongest anxiety med, but minimal risks or side effects

Drug Class: Anxiolytic (anxiety medication): 5-HT1A serotonin receptor partial agonist

➤ 5-HT = serotonin

➤ 5-HT1A = the first serotonin receptor by name

➤ A partial agonist stimulates a receptor, but less strongly than an agonist (serotonin)

Similar Drugs: Hydroxyzine (#46) – non-controlled anxiety med with different mechanism **Comparisons:** Buspirone takes weeks to work, compared to ~ 1 hr with hydroxyzine; Hydroxyzine causes sedation and acts as an antihistamine; Buspirone is non-sedating and works on serotonin receptors; Unlike benzos, buspirone does not cause addiction or withdrawal

Controlled Substance: ✅ Not controlled

High-Alert Risk: ✅ Not high alert; Does not cause serotonin toxicity – ok to combine with antidepressants

Major Side Effects: Minimal side effects, although dizziness, headache, and nausea are possible

Look-Alike/Sound-Alike: Bupropion

Narrow Therapeutic Index: ✅ Wide therapeutic index – not deadly even in large overdose **Precautions:** Not effective for acute anxiety or panic; Takes 2–4 weeks for full effect

Routes: Oral

Easily Replaceable? Partially – some antidepressants and antipsychotics have 5-HT1A effects; OTC lavender extract (CalmAid) has a similar mechanism

Sample Test Questions:

Q: Is buspirone sedating like benzodiazepines and hydroxyzine?

A: No

Q: How long does buspirone take to work?

A: 2–4 weeks

Q: Is buspirone a controlled substance?

A: No

#55 Tramadol (ULTRAM)

TRA-ma-dol (ULL-tram)
Common Uses: Moderate pain
Mascot: "Ultra-ram Trauma doll"

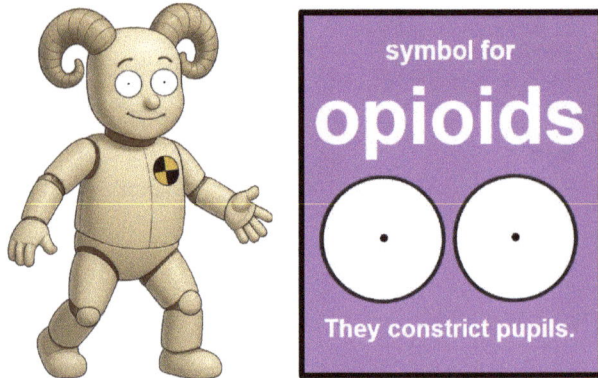

symbol for
opioids
They constrict pupils.

Alternate Mnemonics:

❖ "Tram travels dual track" – opioid and SNRI

❖ "Tramadol dulls pain"

Drug Class: Analgesic (pain med): weak opioid + serotonin and norepinephrine reuptake inhibitor (SNRI)
Similar Drugs: None
Comparisons: Weaker than full opioids; Similar effects to SNRI antidepressants like Duloxetine (#31), Venlafaxine (#44), Desvenlafaxine (#208)
Controlled Substance: ⚠ C-IV (Schedule IV) → Lower abuse risk than full opioids, which are C-II
High-Alert Risk: ⚠ ⚠ Risk of seizures and addiction

➤ Serotonin toxicity – dangerous if combined with a monoamine oxidase inhibitor (MAOI) – phenelzine, tranylcypromine, isocarboxazid, selegiline, linezolid, or methylene blue
Major Side Effects: Dizziness, nausea, constipation, sedation
Look-Alike/Sound-Alike: Trazodone
Narrow Therapeutic Index: No
Precautions: Avoid if seizure disorder; Avoid with serotonin reuptake inhibitors (SSRIs, SNRIs, other antidepressants) to avoid (non-life threatening) serotonin toxicity symptoms such as twitching and sweating
Easily Replaceable? Yes – although with two separate products: low-dose opioid + SNRI

Sample Test Questions:
Q: What schedule is tramadol?
A: C-IV – less strictly controlled than C-II opioids
Q: What neurotransmitters does tramadol affect?
A: Serotonin and norepinephrine

#56 Empagliflozin (JARDIANCE)

em-pa-GLIF-loe-zin (JAR-dee-ance)
Common Uses: Type 2 diabetes, heart failure, chronic kidney disease (CKD)
Mascot: "Empty Jar dance"

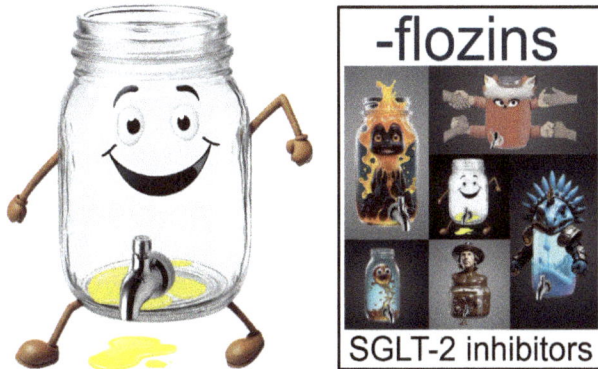

-flozins
SGLT-2 inhibitors

Alternate Mnemonics:

❖ "SGLT2 = Sugar Goes out in Little Tubules"

❖ *SGLT-2 Inhibitors* song available on YouTube, Spotify, etc

Drug Class: Antidiabetic: SGLT2 inhibitor
Similar Drugs: Dapagliflozin (#115), Canagliflozin (>#300)
Comparisons: Strongest evidence for cardiovascular mortality reduction among SGLT2 inhibitors
High-Alert Risk: ⚠ Serious genital infections, rare ketoacidosis (acid buildup from fat breakdown)
Major Side Effects: Genital yeast infections, volume depletion
Look-Alike/Sound-Alike: Jardiance vs. Janumet
Narrow Therapeutic Index: No
Precautions: Monitor for dehydration and ketoacidosis (nausea, fruity breath, rapid breathing)
Routes: Oral
Easily Replaceable? Yes – other SGLT2 inhibitors are comparable

Sample Test Questions:
Q: What class is empagliflozin?
A: SGLT2 inhibitor
Q: How does empagliflozin lower glucose?
A: Increases urinary glucose excretion
Q: What infection is a known side effect of SGLT2 inhibitors?
A: Genital yeast infection
Q: What else is empagliflozin used for besides diabetes?
A: Heart failure and kidney disease

#57 Clonazepam (KLONOPIN)

kloe-NAZ-eh-pam (KLON-oh-pin)
Common Uses: Benzodiazepine (benzo) for anxiety, seizures
Mascot: "Cloned pins"

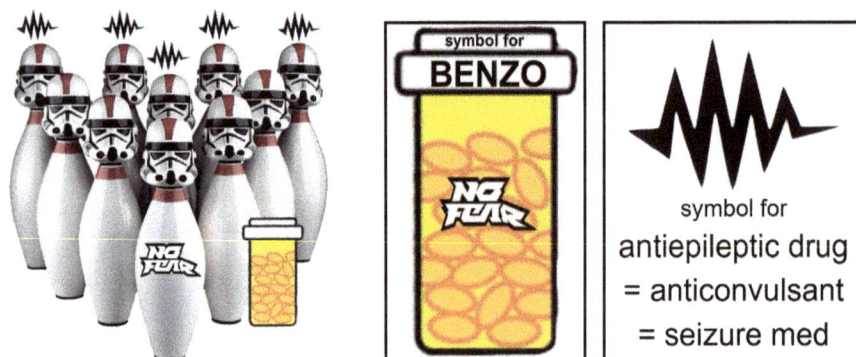

Alternate Mnemonics:

❖ "Klonopin = clone o' calm"

Drug Class: Anxiolytic (anxiety medication) / Anticonvulsant: Benzodiazepine
Similar Drugs: Diazepam (#169), Lorazepam (#81), Alprazolam (#41)
Comparisons: Slower onset and longer duration of effect than alprazolam (Xanax)
Controlled Substance: ⚠ C-IV (Schedule IV) – like other benzos
High-Alert Risk: ⚠ ⚠ ⚠ Risk of respiratory depression, falls, and dependence
Major Side Effects: Drowsiness, dizziness, ataxia, dependence
Look-Alike/Sound-Alike: Clonidine, Clozapine
Narrow Therapeutic Index: No
Precautions:

➤ Avoid with alcohol or opioids – risk of respiratory depression and death

➤ Avoid abrupt discontinuation due to potentially dangerous withdrawal with seizures

➤ Potentially hazardous in older adults – falls, may accumulate due to long half-life

Routes: Oral
Easily Replaceable? Yes – dose conversions defined with other benzos
Also: Benzo withdrawal is nearly identical to alcohol withdrawal

Sample Test Questions:
Q: What class is clonazepam?
A: Benzodiazepine
Q: What is a common risk of abrupt benzo withdrawal?
A: Seizures
Q: What schedule is clonazepam?
A: C-IV (Schedule IV) – like all benzos

#58 Lamotrigine (LAMICTAL)

la-MOE-trih-jeen (LAM-ik-tal)
Common Uses: Bipolar disorder, epilepsy
Mascot: "Ictal Lamb" – Ictal means "having a seizure"

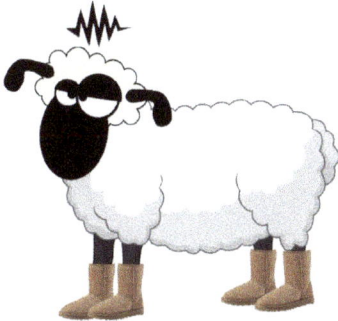

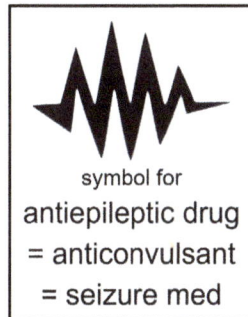

symbol for
antiepileptic drug
= anticonvulsant
= seizure med

Alternate Mnemonics:

❖ "LAM = Less Affective Madness" – Affective relates to mood – used for bipolar disorder
Drug Class: Anticonvulsant/Mood stabilizer: Sodium channel blocker
Similar Drugs: Topiramate (#84), Valproate (#174), Levetiracetam (#123), Lithium (#212)
Comparisons: The fewest side effects of any medication for bipolar disorder; Also the slowest to reach an effective dose (must be increased over weeks to avoid dangerous rash)
Controlled Substance: ✅ Not controlled
High-Alert Risk: ⚠️ ⚠️ ⚠️ Stevens-Johnson Syndrome (life-threatening rash) with rapid dose escalation
Major Side Effects: Rash (usually benign but may be dangerous); At high dose: dizziness, double vision
Look-Alike/Sound-Alike: Lamisil
Narrow Therapeutic Index: No
Precautions: Titrate slowly over several weeks to avoid rash; Discontinue if rash develops
Routes: Oral
Easily Replaceable? No – lamotrigine has unique properties
Also: The antiepileptic (seizure medication) preferred during pregnancy

Sample Test Questions:
Q: What is lamotrigine used for in psychiatry?
A: Bipolar disorder
Q: What serious skin condition is a known risk?
A: Stevens-Johnson Syndrome (SJS)
Q: Why must lamotrigine be titrated slowly?
A: To reduce risk of SJS
Q: Among medications for bipolar disorder and epilepsy, what is the advantage of lamotrigine?
A: Fewer side effects

#59 Fluticasone + Salmeterol (ADVAIR)

floo-TIK-a-sone; sal-MEH-te-role (ADD-vair)
Common Uses: Asthma, Chronic Obstructive Pulmonary Disease (COPD)
Mascot: "Flo's ventilated Flute case" (FLOVENT #25) + "Salamander meter Servant" (SEREVENT >#300)

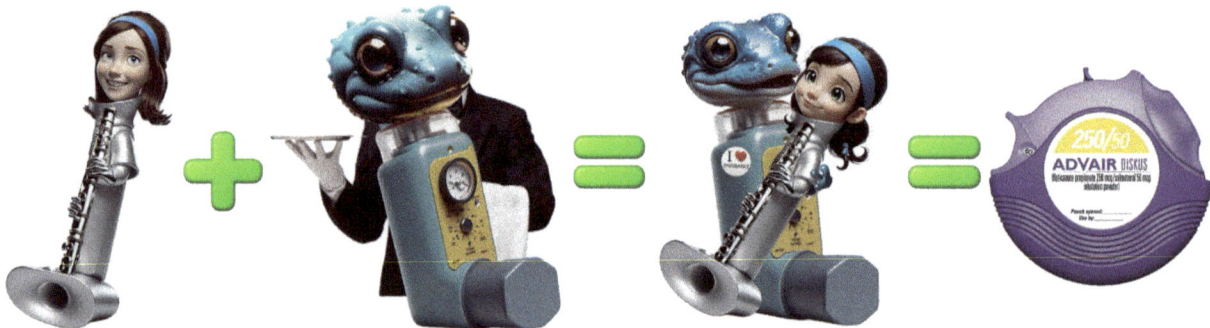

Alternate Mnemonics:

❖ "Fluti + Salm = flare stopper team"

❖ "Advair adds air"

Drug Class: Respiratory: Inhaled corticosteroid + long-acting beta agonist (ICS + LABA)
Similar Drugs: Budesonide/Formoterol (#83), Fluticasone/Vilanterol (#145)
Comparisons: Salmeterol is slower than formoterol; not for acute relief
High-Alert Risk: ✅ Not high alert
Major Side Effects: Thrush (yeast infection of mouth or throat), cough, tremor, hoarseness
Look-Alike/Sound-Alike: Advicor, Advil
Narrow Therapeutic Index: No
Precautions:

➤ Rinse mouth after use to prevent thrush

➤ Not a rescue inhaler for acute asthma attacks

Routes: Inhalation
Easily Replaceable? Yes – other ICS + LABA combos are comparable
Also: Advair Diskus (dry powder, shown above) and Advair HFA (metered-dose inhaler) are not interchangeable

Sample Test Questions:
Q: What does fluticasone do?
A: Reduces airway inflammation
Q: What's the role of salmeterol in Advair?
A: Long-acting bronchodilator
Q: Why rinse after inhaler use?
A: To prevent oral thrush (from fluticasone)
Q: Is Advair for acute asthma attacks?
A: No

#60 Oxycodone (ROXICODONE, OXYCONTIN)

OX-ee-koe-dohn (ROX-ee-koe-dohn, OX-ee-con-tin)

Common Uses: Moderate to severe pain

Mascot: "Perky Ox coding"

➤ She's a "Perky Ox coding" because oxycodone + acetaminophen = PERCOCET (#98)

➤ "Oxycotton tail" for Oxycontin → the mascot has a bunny tail

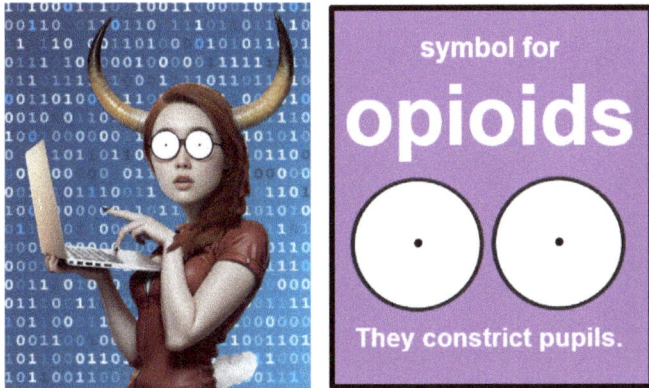

symbol for
opioids

They constrict pupils.

Alternate Mnemonics:

❖ OxyCONTIN is the Controlled Release (CR) form → "CONTINuous Oxy" – taken every 12 hours

❖ "Roxicodone rocks you quick" – the Immediate Release (IR) form – lasts 4 to 6 hours

❖ Songs *The Holy Trinity: Carisoprodol, Alprazolam & Oxycodone* and *Allergic to Everything but Oxy* on YouTube, Spotify, etc

Drug Class: Opioid analgesic: Mu-opioid receptor agonist

Similar Drugs: Hydrocodone/APAP (#23), Oxycodone/APAP (#98), Morphine (#140)

Comparisons: Stronger than codeine or hydrocodone; higher abuse potential (especially IR form)

Controlled Substance: ⚠ ⚠ ⚠ C-II (Schedule II) – like most opioids

High-Alert Risk: ⚠ ⚠ ⚠ ⚠ – high risk for misuse, addiction, respiratory depression, fatal overdose

Major Side Effects: Constipation, sedation, nausea

Look-Alike/Sound-Alike: Oxybutynin, oxytocin

Narrow Therapeutic Index: ⚠ Yes – respiratory depression with opioids

Precautions: Avoid with alcohol or benzodiazepines (↑ fatality risk); Taper to avoid withdrawal

Routes: Oral

Easily Replaceable? Yes – other opioids are comparable with defined dose conversions

Also: The so-called "Holy Trinity" is a dangerous combo of oxycodone + alprazolam (Xanax) + carisoprodol (Soma, a muscle relaxant), as described in the Netflix docuseries *The Pharmacist.*

Sample Test Questions:

Q: What's the most serious risk with oxycodone?

A: Respiratory depression → death

#61 Ondansetron (ZOFRAN)

on-DAN-se-tron (ZOH-fran)
Common Uses: Nausea and vomiting
Mascot: "On Dancer Tron! (Go) so frantic!"

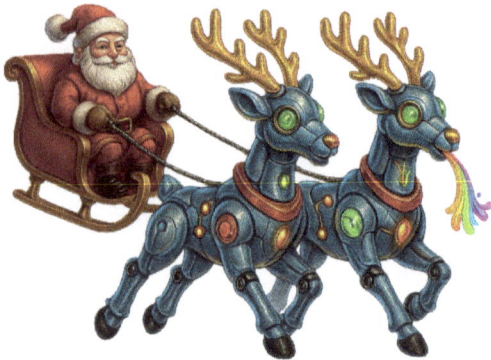

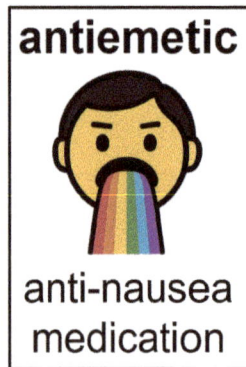
antiemetic
anti-nausea medication

Alternate Mnemonics:

❖ "Zofran zaps nausea"

❖ "Zofran = zero fran(tic) barfing"

❖ "Setron = serotonin stop"

Drug Class: Antiemetic: 5-HT3 serotonin receptor antagonist
Similar Drugs: Granisetron (>#300), Dolasetron (>#300), Palonosetron (>#300)
Comparisons: More effective than promethazine (#198) and less sedating
Controlled Substance: ✅ Not controlled
High-Alert Risk: ✅ Not high alert
Major Side Effects: Constipation, QT prolongation (slowed cardiac conduction), dizziness, headache
Look-Alike/Sound-Alike: Zoloft
Narrow Therapeutic Index: ⚠ Risk of QT prolongation at high doses or intravenous form
Routes: Oral, IV
Easily Replaceable? Yes – other antiemetics may be used; Other -setron antiemetics are expensive
Also: Orally disintegrating tablet (ODT) is often used; Does not cause serotonin toxicity (it blocks rather than stimulates a serotonin receptor)

Sample Test Questions:
Q: What type of receptor does ondansetron block?
A: Serotonin receptor (5-HT3)
Q: What's a cardiac side effect of ondansetron?
A: QT prolongation

#62 Cholecalciferol (VITAMIN D3)

KOH-leh-KAL-sih-fer-ol (VY-tuh-min DEE three)

Common Uses: Vitamin D deficiency, osteoporosis prevention

Mascot: "Cholesterol Calcium for All"

➤ Derived from cholesterol, synthesized in the skin via sunlight – beach has a "fatty" appearance

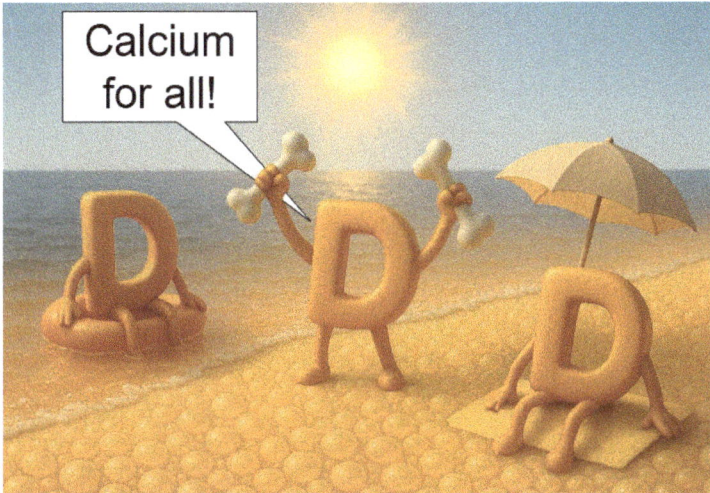

Alternate Mnemonics:

❖ "Sunny-D3"

Drug Class: Supplement: Vitamin D analog

Similar Drugs: Ergocalciferol (#38), Calcitriol (#254)

Comparisons: D3 (cholecalciferol) is better absorbed than D2 (ergocalciferol)

High-Alert Risk: ✅ Not high alert

Major Side Effects: Rare hypercalcemia (high calcium)

Look-Alike/Sound-Alike: Cholestyramine

Narrow Therapeutic Index: No

Precautions: Avoid megadoses without medical supervision

Routes: Oral

Easily Replaceable? Yes – other vitamin D analogs are comparable

Also: Available over-the-counter (OTC); Activated first in the liver, then in the kidneys to form calcitriol

Sample Test Questions:

Q: What is the active form of cholecalciferol?

A: Calcitriol

Q: What mineral does vitamin D help absorb?

A: Calcium

Q: What's the preferred vitamin D supplement?

A: D3 (cholecalciferol)

#63 Atenolol (TENORMIN)

uh-TEN-oh-lol (ten-OR-min)

Common uses: High blood pressure, angina (cardiac chest pain), post-heart attack

Mascot: "A tin Tenor man"

➤ Like other beta blocker mascots, he wears a 'LOL' hat with prongs marked β

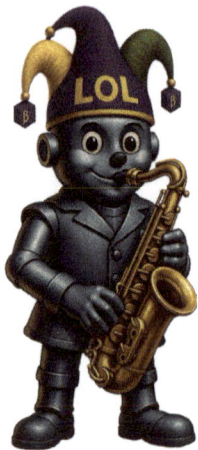

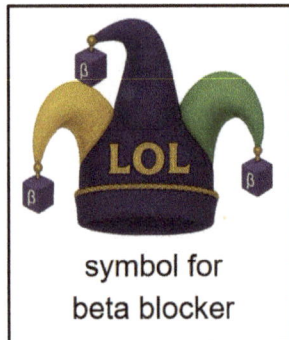

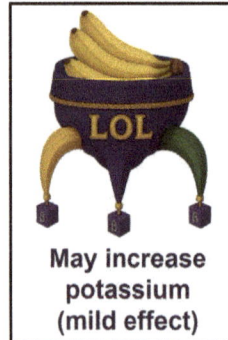

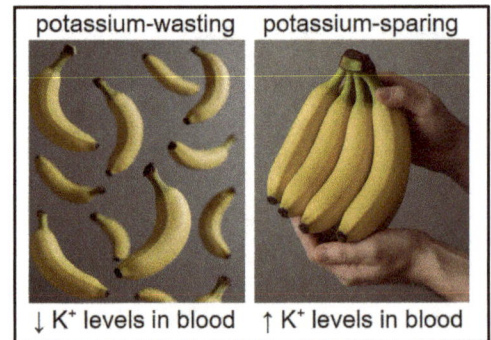

symbol for
beta blocker

May increase
potassium
(mild effect)

potassium-wasting   potassium-sparing

↓ K⁺ levels in blood   ↑ K⁺ levels in blood

Alternate Mnemonics:

❖ "Atenolol = attend to heart rate"

❖ "Tenno keeps pressure low and heart rate slow"

Drug Class: Antihypertensive: Beta-1 selective beta blocker

Similar Drugs: Metoprolol (#6), Propranolol (#77), Bisoprolol (#249)

Comparisons: Longer duration of effect allowing once-daily dosing; Unlike propranolol, atenolol does not cross blood-brain barrier; Cleared by kidneys → unlike many others, atenolol requires dose adjustment in kidney disease; Atenolol is not used in heart failure (unlike carvedilol, metoprolol)

High-Alert Risk: ✅ Not high alert

Major Side Effects: Bradycardia (slow heart rate), hypotension (low blood pressure), fatigue

Look-Alike/Sound-Alike: Atorvastatin, Alteplase, Amiodarone

Precautions: Do not stop abruptly; Adjust dose in renal impairment; Use caution in asthma despite β1 selectivity

Routes: Oral

Easily Replaceable? Yes – other beta blockers are comparable

Sample Test Questions:

Q: Why should atenolol not be stopped suddenly?

A: Risk of rebound angina, tachycardia (fast heart rate), or heart attack

Q: How does atenolol differ from propranolol?

A: Atenolol is cardioselective and does not cross the blood-brain barrier

#64 Glimepiride (AMARYL)

GLYE-meh-pir-ide (AM-ah-rill)
Common Uses: Type 2 diabetes
Mascot: "Amarilla Gleeful emperor ride"

➤ Amarilla – spanish for yellow

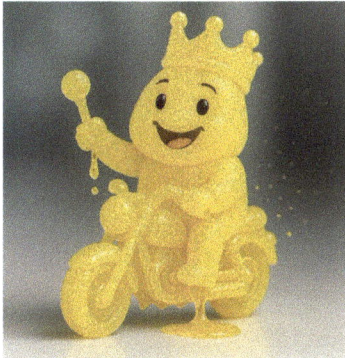

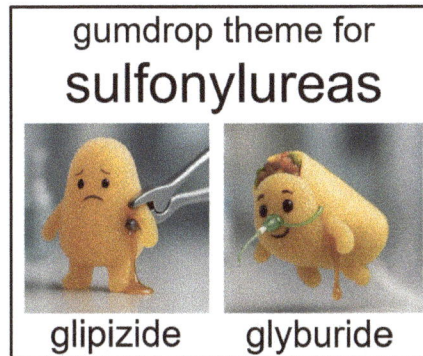

gumdrop theme for **sulfonylureas**
glipizide   glyburide

Alternate Mnemonics:

❖ "Sulfonylurea = stimulates units of insulin"

❖ "Pancreas prodder" → stimulates pancreas directly to secrete insulin regardless of blood sugar

❖ "Glim-glimmer of insulin spark" → ineffective after the pancreas stops making insulin

❖ *Glimepiride* song available on YouTube, Spotify, etc

Drug Class: Antidiabetic: Sulfonylurea
Similar Drugs: Glipizide (#42), Glyburide (>#300)
Comparisons: Longer-acting than glipizide → higher risk of hypoglycemia in elderly
High-Alert Risk: ⚠️ ⚠️ Can cause severe hypoglycemia, especially in elderly or kidney impairment
Major Side Effects: Hypoglycemia (low blood sugar), weight gain, rash
Look-Alike/Sound-Alike: Glipizide
Narrow Therapeutic Index: No
Precautions: Avoid in elderly or those prone to low blood sugar; Take with breakfast
Routes: Oral
Easily Replaceable? Yes – other sulfonylureas are comparable
Also: Most sulfa-allergic patients can take sulfonylureas, but check if the allergy was severe.

Sample Test Questions:
Q: What is a major risk of glimepiride?
A: Hypoglycemia (low blood sugar)
Q: When should glimepiride be taken?
A: With breakfast
Q: Does glimepiride cause weight loss or gain?
A: Weight gain

#65 Folic Acid (VITAMIN B9)

FOE-lik ASS-id

Common Uses: Prevent birth defects, treat folate deficiency

Mascot: "Benign Foliage"

➤ Nine B characters in foliage

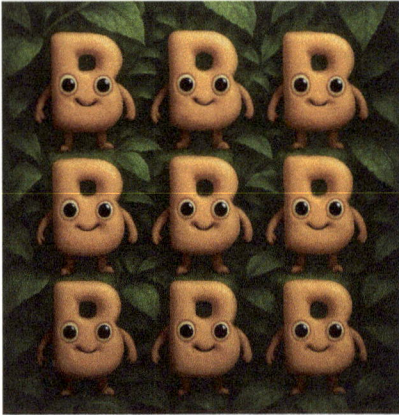

Alternate Mnemonics:

❖ "Folic = foliage for fetal spine" → necessary to prevent birth defects (neural tube defects)

Drug Class: Vitamin supplement

Similar Drugs: Cyanocobalamin (#131) is Vitamin B12

Comparisons: Often used with B12; deficiency overlaps

High-Alert Risk: ✅ Not high alert

Major Side Effects: None expected

Look-Alike/Sound-Alike: Folinic acid (leucovorin)

Narrow Therapeutic Index: No

Precautions: May "mask Vitamin B12 deficiency" by correcting anemia from B12 deficiency, but nerve damage may still worsen unseen

Routes: Oral, IV

Easily Replaceable? Yes – generics and OTC formulations are interchangeable

Also: Required in all women of childbearing age to prevent birth defects; Low B9 levels may worsen depression or reduce antidepressant response

Sample Test Questions:

Q: Should all pregnant women take folic acid?

A: Yes

Q: What birth defect does folic acid prevent?

A: Neural tube defects

Q: Can folic acid mask other deficiencies?

A: Yes – can mask B12 deficiency

Q: Is folic acid available over-the-counter (OTC)?

A: Yes

#66 Zolpidem (AMBIEN)

ZOLE-pih-dem (AM-bee-en)
Common Uses: Insomnia
Mascot: "Amnesia bean Soul pie"

➤ Z's in his eyes because it is a Z-drug (non-benzo sleep aid)

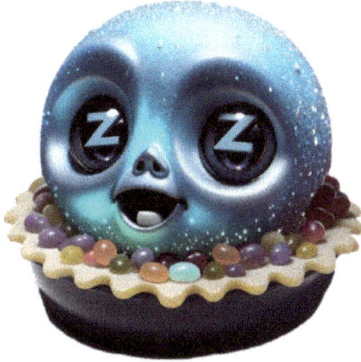

Alternate Mnemonics:
❖ "AMbien, Z-drug = Zzz-until A.M."
Drug Class: Sedative-hypnotic: Non-benzodiazepine GABA-A agonist ("Z-drug")
Similar Drugs: Eszopiclone (>#300), Temazepam (>#300)
Comparisons: Mechanism is similar to benzos; Shorter half-life than benzos; fewer hangover effects
Controlled Substance: ⚠ C-IV (Schedule IV) – same schedule as benzos

➤ Lower abuse potential than benzos but controlled due to misuse and dependence risk

High-Alert Risk: ⚠ ⚠ Risk of sedation, sleepwalking, and complex sleep behaviors

➤ Sleep driving has occurred; Risk of injury while sleepwalking

Major Side Effects: Drowsiness, dizziness, sleepwalking, rebound insomnia
Look-Alike/Sound-Alike: Zoloft, Zaleplon
Narrow Therapeutic Index: No, but high risk of driving impairment if exceeding the recommended dose
Precautions: Avoid alcohol and other CNS depressants; Take right before bed on empty stomach
Routes: Oral
Easily Replaceable? Yes – other sedative-hypnotics are comparable
Also: Female patients require lower doses due to slower clearance

Sample Test Questions:
Q: What class is zolpidem?
A: Sedative-hypnotic ("Z-drug")
Q: What DEA schedule is Ambien?
A: C-IV (Schedule IV) – same as benzos
Q: What serious side effect may occur while asleep?
A: Sleepwalking or sleep driving

#67 Latanoprost (XALATAN)

la-TA-na-prost (ZAL-a-tan)

Common Uses: Glaucoma, ocular hypertension

➤ Glaucoma is eye disease where high pressure damages the optic nerve, risking vision loss

Mascot: "X-tra Latin prost drops"

➤ "Prost" refers to prostaglandin – natural chemical that ↑ fluid drainage from the eye to ↓ pressure

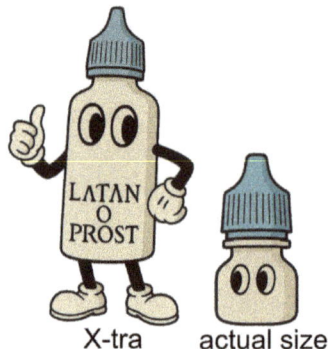

X-tra   actual size

Alternate Mnemonics:

❖ "Latanoprost lets fluid out"

❖ "Xalatan = exit aqueous" – helps lower eye pressure by draining aqueous humor (eye fluid)

Drug Class: Ophthalmic: Prostaglandin analog

Similar Drugs: Bimatoprost (#195), Travoprost (>#300)

Comparisons: Once-daily dosing; more iris darkening than beta blocker eye drops like timolol

High-Alert Risk: Not high alert but may cause irreversible iris color change

Major Side Effects: Eye redness, iris darkening, eyelash growth, blurry vision

Look-Alike/Sound-Alike: Latanoprostene

Narrow Therapeutic Index: No

Precautions: Store unopened bottles in refrigerator

Routes: Ophthalmic

Easily Replaceable? Yes – other prostaglandin analogs are comparable

Also: Once-daily dosing at bedtime preferred

Sample Test Questions:

Q: What does latanoprost treat?

A: Glaucoma

Q: What class is latanoprost?

A: Prostaglandin analog

Q: What unusual side effect may occur?

A: Iris color change and eyelash growth

Q: How is latanoprost stored?

A: Unopened bottles in the fridge

#68 Doxycycline (VIBRAMYCIN)

dox-ee-SYE-kleen (VYE-bruh-my-sin)

Common Uses: Acne and infections including pneumonia, Sexually transmitted infections (STIs), Lyme disease

Mascot: "Vibrating Docked cyclone"

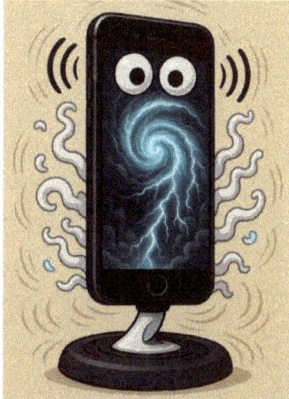

Drug Class: Antibiotic: Tetracycline

Similar Drugs: Minocycline (#269), Tetracycline (>#300)

Comparisons: Better absorption and fewer gastrointestinal (GI) side effects than tetracycline

High-Alert Risk: Not high risk, but may cause esophagitis and photosensitivity reactions

Major Side Effects: GI upset, photosensitivity, esophagitis, tooth discoloration

Look-Alike/Sound-Alike: Doxepin

Narrow Therapeutic Index: No

Precautions:

➤ Remain upright after dosing to prevent esophagitis

➤ Avoid in children <8 due to tooth discoloration

Routes: Oral, IV

Easily Replaceable? Yes – other tetracyclines are comparable

Also: Avoid dairy within 1–2 hours of dosing – calcium blocks absorption of doxycycline

Sample Test Questions:

Q: What class is doxycycline?

A: Tetracycline antibiotic

Q: What side effect of doxycycline involves sun exposure?

A: Photosensitivity

Q: Why should doxycycline be avoided in children under age 8?

A: Tooth discoloration

Q: How should doxycycline be taken to avoid inflammation of the esophagus?

A: With water and remain upright

#69 Lisdexamfetamine (VYVANSE)

lis-DEX-am-fet-a-meen (VYE-vanss)

Common Uses: ADHD, binge eating disorder

Mascot: "Lis decks amp with feta to reVive Vance"

This one's busy, but bear with me... This is the only amphetamine spelled "fet" (like feta cheese) instead of "phet". Vyvanse is "revived" – activated actually – in the red blood cells. This makes the medication last longer with slower/smoother onset, and also serves as an abuse deterrent. Injection of Vyvanse does not cause immediate euphoria because the drug needs to be activated in RBCs first. Despite being less abusable, Vyvanse is still a Schedule II controlled substance, like Adderall.

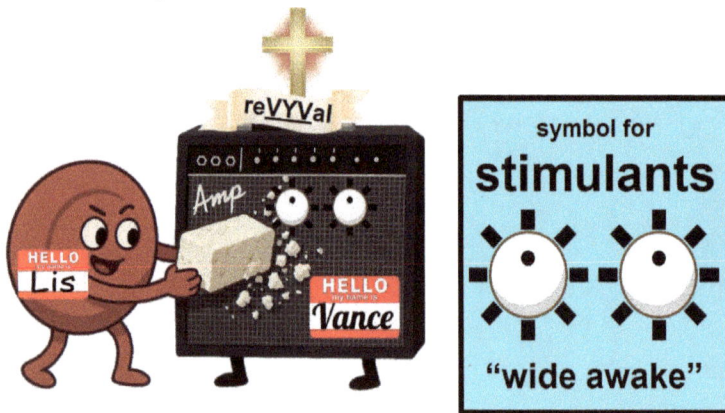

Alternate Mnemonics:

- ❖ "Lis = leash on dexamphetamine" – "leashed dextroamphetamine"
- ❖ "Long leash, long action"
- ❖ "Once-daily leash release"

Drug Class: CNS stimulant: Amphetamine

Similar Drugs: Concerta – long-acting methylphenidate (#32), Extended-release Adderall (#14)

Comparisons: Longer onset, smoother duration than immediate-release stimulants

Controlled Substance: ⚠ ⚠ ⚠ C-II (Schedule II) – like other amphetamine products

High-Alert Risk: ⚠ But lower risk of misuse than immediate-release amphetamine products

Major Side Effects: Appetite loss, insomnia, irritability, increased heart rate

Look-Alike/Sound-Alike: Lisinopril

Narrow Therapeutic Index: No

Precautions: Monitor BP, HR, and growth in children

Routes: Oral

Easily Replaceable? Partially – other stimulants are similar, but response varies

Also: Unlike most extended-release capsules, Vyvanse capsules can be opened and contents sprinkled on food

Sample Test Questions:

Q: What is lisdexamfetamine converted to in red blood cells?

A: Dextroamphetamine

#70 Insulin Lispro (HUMALOG)

IN-su-lin LISS-pro (HYOO-mah-log)
Common Uses: Mealtime insulin for Type 1 and Type 2 diabetes
Mascot: "Hum a log with a Lisp"

➤ Nearly identical to the other '-log' insulin: insulin aspart (NOVOLOG)

◇ Think dinner plate when you see the "log" in the mascot images for HUMALOG & NOVOLOG

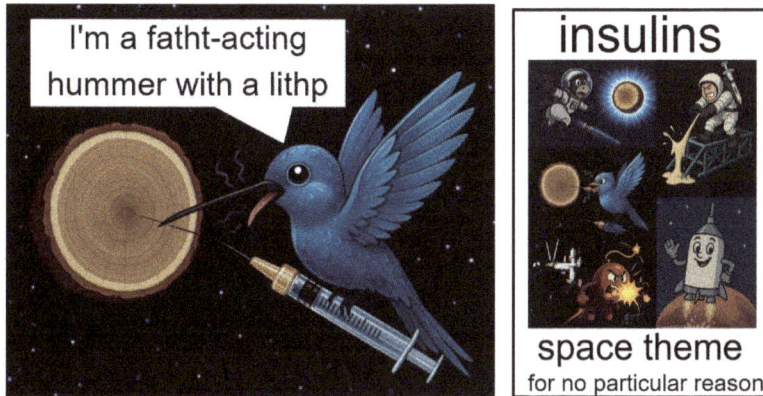

Alternate Mnemonics:

❖ Take with meals: "Lispro with lasagna, lentils, etc."

Drug Class: Antidiabetic: Rapid-acting mealtime insulin
Similar Drugs: Insulin Aspart (#76), Insulin Glulisine (>#300)
Comparisons: Nearly identical to insulin aspart; Onset within 15 min; shorter duration than regular insulin
High-Alert Risk: ⚠ ⚠ ⚠ ⚠ High risk of hypoglycemia (low blood sugar) if dosed incorrectly
Major Side Effects: Hypoglycemia, weight gain, injection site reaction
Look-Alike/Sound-Alike: Humalog vs. Humulin
Narrow Therapeutic Index: ⚠ ⚠ ⚠ Yes – Narrow Therapeutic Index
Precautions:

➤ Dose closely timed with meals

➤ Rotate injection sites to avoid lipodystrophy (abnormal fat loss or buildup)

Routes: Subcutaneous (SubQ)
Easily Replaceable? Yes – other rapid insulins are comparable

Sample Test Questions:
Q: What kind of insulin is lispro?
A: Rapid-acting
Q: When should lispro be given?
A: Within 15 minutes of eating
Q: What is the most dangerous side effect?
A: Hypoglycemia

#71 Clonidine (CATAPRES)

KLON-ih-deen (KAT-uh-press)

Common Uses: Hypertension, ADHD, aggressive behavior, opioid withdrawal, tics, insomnia

Mascot: "Clown dines → Cat impressed"

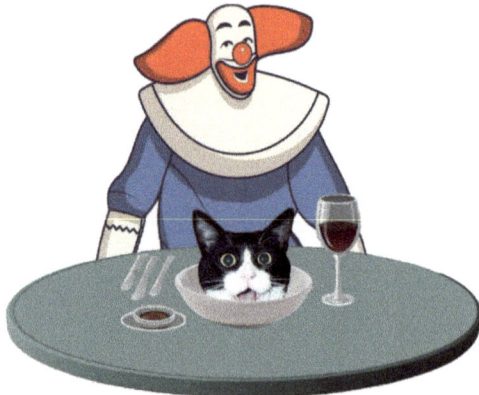

Alternate Mnemonics:

❖ "Catapres = cat presses down BP" or "Cat Alpha press" for α2 receptor activator

❖ "Press pause on pressure"

Drug Class: Antihypertensive: Alpha-2 adrenergic agonist

➤ Activates Alpha-2 receptors in the brain, which are a type of receptor for norepinephrine

Similar Drugs: Guanfacine (#275)

Comparisons: One of two antihypertensives (blood pressure meds) used for ADHD (also guanfacine); Clonidine is more sedating than most antihypertensives, including guanfacine

Controlled Substance: ✅ Not controlled

High-Alert Risk: ⚠️ ⚠️ Risk of rebound hypertension if stopped suddenly

Major Side Effects: Drowsiness, dry mouth, bradycardia (slow heart rate)

Look-Alike/Sound-Alike: Klonopin, Clozapine

Narrow Therapeutic Index: Moderate – blood pressure drop

Precautions: Monitor for sedation, especially with other CNS depressants; Do not stop abruptly

Routes: Oral, transdermal patch

Easily Replaceable? Partially – guanfacine is similar, but less sedating

Sample Test Questions:

Q: What receptor does clonidine stimulate?

A: Alpha-2 adrenergic receptors

Q: What happens if clonidine is stopped abruptly?

A: Rebound hypertension

Q: What's a common side effect of clonidine?

A: Sedation

#72 Loratadine (CLARITIN)

lor-AT-uh-deen (KLAIR-ih-tin)
Common Uses: Seasonal allergies, allergic rhinitis (runny nose)
Mascot: "Low rat dines, with Clarity"

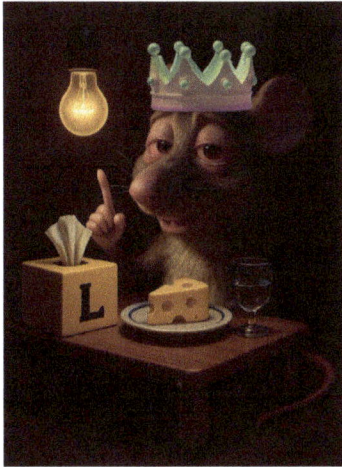

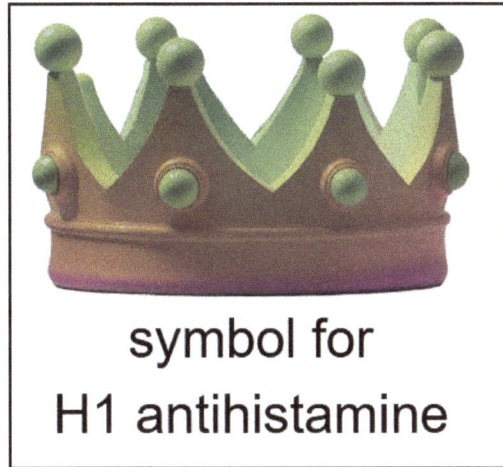

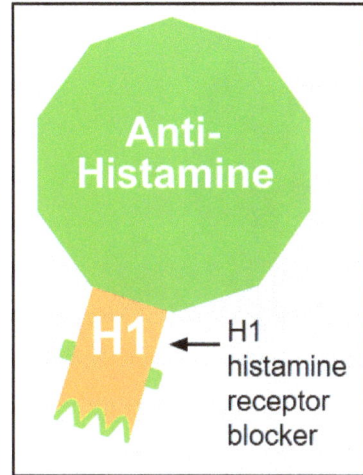

symbol for
H1 antihistamine

Anti-Histamine

H1 ← H1 histamine receptor blocker

Drug Class: Antihistamine: 2nd-generation H1 blocker
Similar Drugs: Cetirizine (#43), Levocetirizine (#152), Fexofenadine (#257)
Comparisons: Less sedating than 1st-gen antihistamines like diphenhydramine (Benadryl)
High-Alert Risk: ☑ Not high alert
Major Side Effects: None expected, sedation rarely
Look-Alike/Sound-Alike: Clarinex
Narrow Therapeutic Index: ☑ No – It has a wide therapeutic index
Precautions: None – safe at standard doses
Routes: Oral
Easily Replaceable? Yes – other second-gen antihistamines are comparable
Also: Take daily during allergy season for prevention; Available OTC and in combo with pseudoephedrine

Sample Test Questions:
Q: What class is loratadine?
A: 2nd-generation antihistamine
Q: Does loratadine cause sedation?
A: Rarely – much less than older antihistamines
Q: Is loratadine available over-the-counter?
A: Yes
Q: What symptom does loratadine treat?
A: Seasonal allergies

#73 Finasteride (PROPECIA, PROSCAR)

fin-AS-tur-ide (pro-PEE-sha, PRO-skar)

Common Uses: Benign prostatic hyperplasia (BPH, enlarged prostate), male pattern hair loss

Mascot: "Finn Asteroid's Prostate scare"

➤ Finn from *Adventure Time* dreads a prostate exam

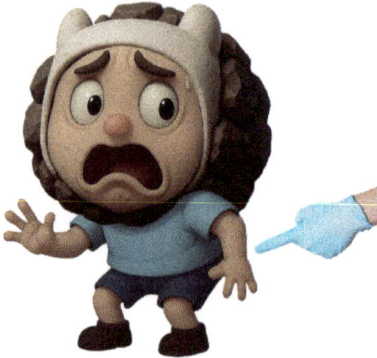

Alternate Mnemonics:

❖ "Fin = finishes Dihydrotestosterone (DHT)"

❖ "Propecia protects your precious hair"

Drug Class: Hormone modulator: 5-alpha reductase inhibitor

Similar Drugs: Dutasteride (>#300)

Comparisons: Finasteride is selective for type II enzyme; dutasteride blocks both I & II

High-Alert Risk: ⚠ Teratogenic (risk of birth defects) if handled by pregnant women – due to interference with development of male genitalia

Major Side Effects: Decreased libido, erectile dysfunction, gynecomastia (male breast enlargement), depression

Look-Alike/Sound-Alike: Proscar vs. Provera

Narrow Therapeutic Index: No

Precautions: Women should not handle crushed tablets; May take 6 months to see effect

Routes: Oral

Easily Replaceable? Partially – dutasteride is the closest direct substitute

Sample Test Questions:

Q: What hormone does finasteride inhibit?

A: Dihydrotestosterone (DHT)

Q: What condition is Propecia used for?

A: Male pattern baldness

Q: Who should not handle finasteride?

A: Pregnant women

Q: How long does it take finasteride to work?

A: Up to 6 months

#74 Dulaglutide (TRULICITY)

doo-la-GLOO-tide (troo-LISS-i-tee)
Common Uses: Type 2 diabetes
Mascot: "Truly a Doula"

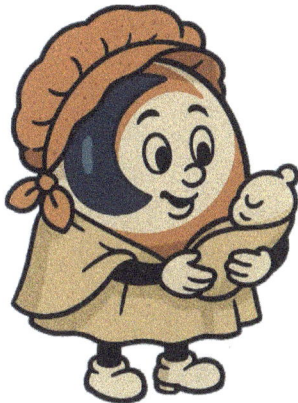

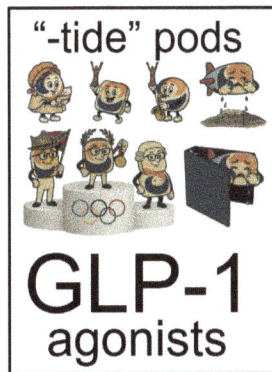

Alternate Mnemonics:
- ❖ "Dula = dual benefit: diabetes + weight"

Drug Class: Antidiabetic: GLP-1 receptor agonist
Similar Drugs: Semaglutide (#48), Liraglutide (#139), Tirzepatide (New)
Comparisons: Once-weekly like semaglutide; Slower weight loss than semaglutide
High-Alert Risk: ⚠️ ⚠️ Risk of thyroid C-cell tumors. tumors, Delayed stomach emptying can lead to aspiration (stomach contents breathed into lungs)
Major Side Effects: Nausea, vomiting, diarrhea, thyroid tumor risk
Look-Alike/Sound-Alike: Trulance
Narrow Therapeutic Index: No
Precautions: Contraindicated with personal/family history of medullary thyroid cancer; Titrate slowly to reduce GI effects; Hold before surgery due to risk of aspiration
Routes: Subcutaneous (SubQ)
Easily Replaceable? Yes – other GLP-1 agonists are comparable

Sample Test Questions:
Q: What class is dulaglutide?
A: GLP-1 receptor agonist
Q: What is Trulicity used for?
A: Type 2 diabetes
Q: How often is dulaglutide injected?
A: Once weekly
Q: Why should GLP-1 agonists be held prior to surgery?
A: To avoid aspiration of stomach contents while under anaesthesia

#75 Hydrochlorothiazide + Losartan (HYZAAR)

hye-droe-klor-oh-THYE-a-zide; loe-SAR-tan

Common Uses: Hypertension

Mascots: "Micro Hydrant, tie-dyed" (#12) + "Cozier Lord sa(r)tan" (#8)

➤ Hydrochlorothiazide (HCTZ) lowers potassium (K+) by causing it to be lost in the urine, while losartan helps retain potassium. Together, their effects balance, keeping K+ levels more stable

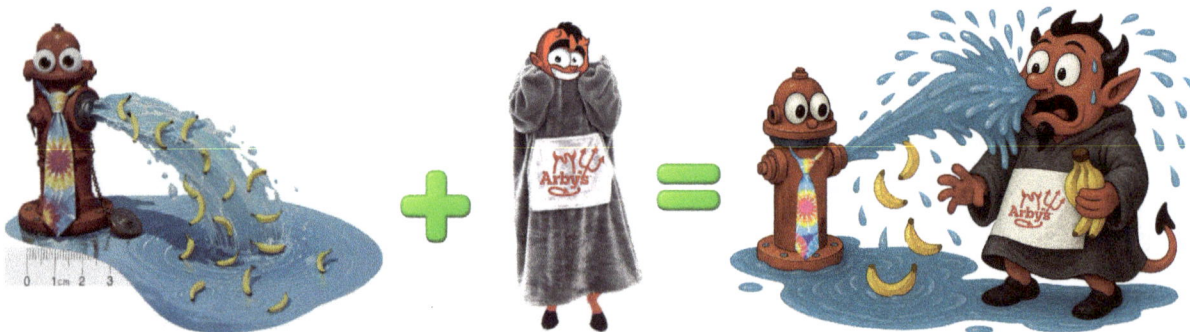

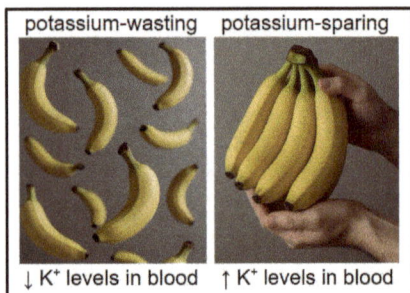

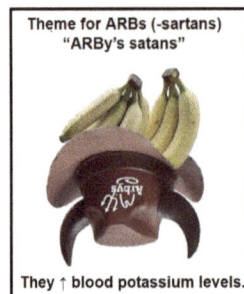

potassium-wasting	potassium-sparing
↓ K+ levels in blood	↑ K+ levels in blood

Theme for ARBs (-sartans)
"ARBy's satans"

They ↑ blood potassium levels.

Drug Class: Antihypertensive: Angiotensin II Receptor Blocker (ARB) + Thiazide diuretic

➤ HCTZ = hydrochlorothiazide

Similar Drugs: Lisinopril/HCTZ (#53), Valsartan/HCTZ (not Top 300), Olmesartan/HCTZ (#235)

Comparisons: ARB + thiazide combos reduce BP via dual mechanism with less cough than ACE combos

High-Alert Risk: ⚠ Risk of hypotension, electrolyte disturbances

Narrow Therapeutic Index: No

Precautions: Avoid in pregnancy; Monitor electrolytes and kidney function

Routes: Oral

Easily Replaceable? Yes – other ARB or ACE inhibitor + HCTZ combos are comparable

Sample Test Questions:

Q: Why is losartan added to HCTZ?

A: Enhance BP-lowering effect and prevent low potassium levels

Q: In HCTZ/losartan combo, which component is the diuretic?

A: HCTZ

#76 Insulin Aspart (NOVOLOG)

IN-su-lin ASS-part (NO-vo-log)

Common Uses: Mealtime insulin for Type 1 and Type 2 diabetes

Mascot: "Nova log (blows) Ass apart"

➤ Nearly identical to fellow '-log' insulin: lispro (HUMALOG)

◇ Think dinner plate when you see the "log" in the mascot images for HUMALOG & NOVOLOG

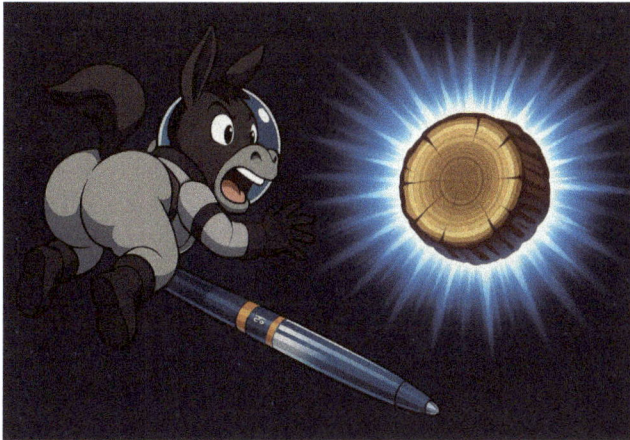

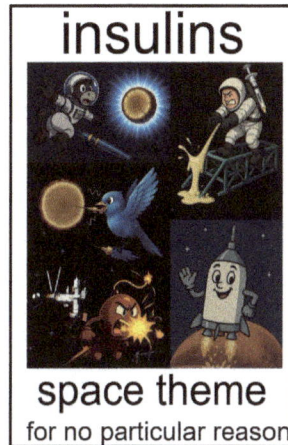

insulins

space theme
for no particular reason

Alternate Mnemonics:

❖ "Aspart = As-part of the meal"

Drug Class: Antidiabetic: Rapid-acting mealtime insulin

Similar Drugs: Insulin Lispro (#70), Insulin Glulisine (#>300)

Comparisons: Nearly identical to insulin lispro; Onset within 15 min; shorter duration than regular insulin

High-Alert Risk: ⚠ ⚠ ⚠ ⚠ High risk of hypoglycemia if dosed incorrectly

Major Side Effects: Hypoglycemia, weight gain, lipodystrophy, injection site reaction

Look-Alike/Sound-Alike: NovoLog vs. NovoLIN

Narrow Therapeutic Index: ⚠ ⚠ ⚠ Yes

Precautions:

➤ Dose closely timed with meals

➤ Rotate injection sites to avoid lipodystrophy (abnormal fat loss or buildup)

Routes: Subcutaneous (SubQ)

Easily Replaceable? Yes – other rapid-acting insulins are comparable

Sample Test Questions:

Q: What should be done to avoid lipodystrophy?

A: Rotate injection sites

Q: When should insulin aspart be given?

A: Just before meals

#77 Propranolol (INDERAL)

pro-PRAN-oh-lol (IN-der-al)

Common Uses: Hypertension, performance anxiety, migraine prevention, arrhythmias, tremors

Mascot: "Ender-Prop ran"

➤ Ender from *Ender's Game* with a propeller arm

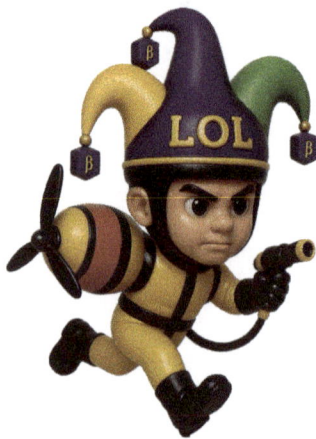

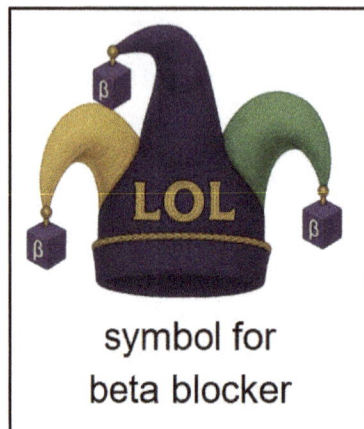

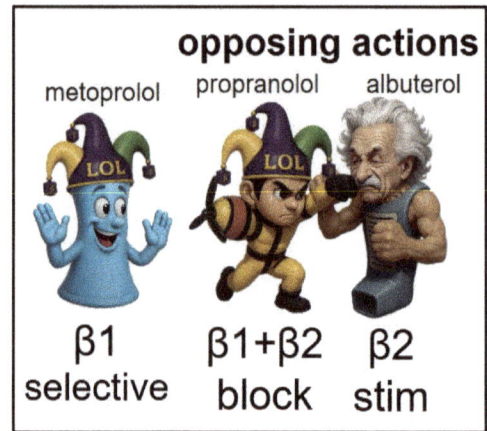

symbol for
beta blocker

opposing actions

metoprolol	propranolol	albuterol
β1 selective	β1+β2 block	β2 stim

Alternate Mnemonics:

❖ "Propranolol = panic-proof performance"

❖ "Inderal = end-all for test-taking anxiety"

Drug Class: Antihypertensive: Nonselective beta blocker (β1 and β2)

Similar Drugs: Atenolol (#63), Metoprolol (#6), Carvedilol (#34)

Comparisons: Propranolol crosses the blood-brain barrier → especially effective for tremor and performance anxiety

Controlled Substance: ✅ Not controlled

High-Alert Risk: ⚠️ ⚠️ Risk of bronchospasm in asthma, bradycardia (slow heart rate), hypotension

Major Side Effects: Fatigue, dizziness

Narrow Therapeutic Index: No

Precautions: Avoid in asthma and COPD; Taper if stopped to avoid rebound symptoms

Routes: Oral, IV

Easily Replaceable? Partially – although other β blockers may be less effective for tremor and performance anxiety

Also: Does not cause drowsiness; Used off-label to reduce test anxiety

Sample Test Questions:

Q: What side effect makes propranolol risky in asthma?

A: Bronchospasm

Q: Why should propranolol be tapered if stopped?

A: To avoid rebound hypertension or anxiety

#78 Azithromycin (ZITHROMAX, Z-PAK)

az-ITH-roe-my-sin (ZITH-roe-max, ZEE-pack)

Common Uses: Respiratory infections, Sexually Transmitted Infection (STIs), traveler's diarrhea

Mascot: "Zippered mice in there, Pak'd to the Max"

> ➤ 6 mice = 6 tabs in a Z-Pak (5-day treatment)

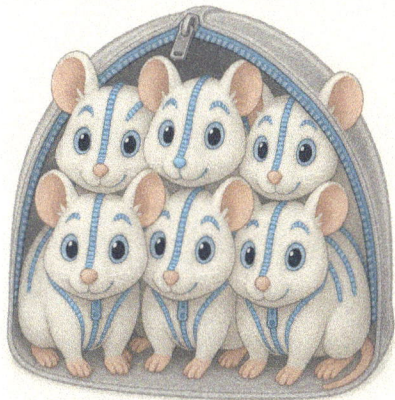

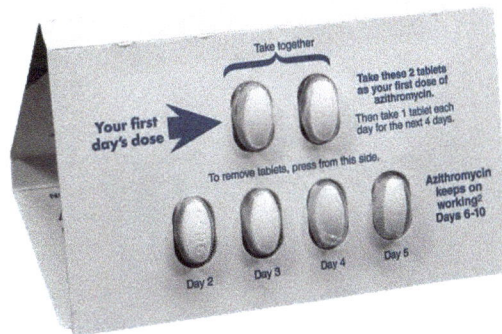

Drug Class: Antibiotic: Macrolide, protein synthesis inhibitor

Similar Drugs: Erythromycin (#271), Clarithromycin (>#300)

Comparisons: Longer half-life and fewer interactions than erythromycin

High-Alert Risk: ⚠ QT prolongation (heart rhythm issue), liver toxicity

Major Side Effects: Diarrhea, nausea, rash

Look-Alike/Sound-Alike: Zyrtec

Narrow Therapeutic Index: No

Precautions: Take on empty stomach if using suspension

Routes: Oral, IV

Easily Replaceable? Yes – other macrolide antibiotics are comparable

Also: Post-antibiotic effect: continues working after last dose

Sample Test Questions:

Q: What class is azithromycin?

A: Macrolide antibiotic

Q: What cardiac risk is associated with azithromycin?

A: QT prolongation

Q: How many days is a Z-pak?

A: 5 days

Q: Is azithromycin a narrow therapeutic index drug?

A: No

#79 Ezetimibe (ZETIA)

eh-ZET-ih-mibe (ZET-ee-uh)

Common Uses: High cholesterol, added to a statin

Mascot: "Easy time for Zeti" = zebra/yeti hybrid dribbling a low density lipoprotein (LDL) – "bad cholesterol"

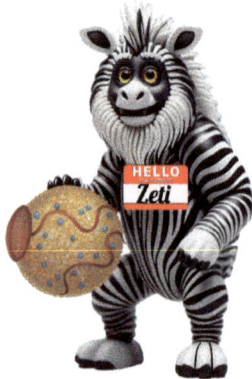

Alternate Mnemonics:

❖ "Easy Time Lowering LDL" – helps reduce cholesterol without much hassle

❖ "Easy Time in the Gut" – works in the intestine, blocking cholesterol absorption

❖ "Easy Time on Side Effects" – fewer risks than statins

❖ "Easy Time Adding On" – to a statin

❖ "Easy Time for the Liver" – minimal liver involvement

Drug Class: Lipid-lowering: Cholesterol absorption inhibitor

Added to Statins: Atorvastatin (#1), Rosuvastatin (#13), Simvastatin (#19)

Comparisons: Unlike statins, ezetimibe does not affect how the liver makes cholesterol; Ezetimibe only works in the intestine; Causes fewer systemic (whole body) side effects than statins

High-Alert Risk: ✅ Not high alert

Major Side Effects: Mild GI upset (e.g., diarrhea, abdominal pain), fatigue

Look-Alike/Sound-Alike: Zestril

Narrow Therapeutic Index: No

Precautions: Not effective alone for high LDL – use with a statin

Routes: Oral

Easily Replaceable? Partially – ezetimibe is the only available drug that specifically blocks the Niemann-Pick C1-Like 1 (NPC1L1) transporter, but other lipid-lowering agents are available

Sample Test Questions:

Q: What does ezetimibe block?

A: Intestinal cholesterol absorption

Q: Is ezetimibe effective when used alone?"

A: Not usually – approved as an add-on to a statin

#80 Ethinyl Estradiol (EE) + Norethindrone (LOESTRIN, MICROGESTIN)

ETH-in-il ESS-truh-dye-ol; nor-ETH-in-drone (LOW-ess-trin, MY-kroh-JESS-tin)

Common Uses: Oral contraception pill (OCP), menstrual regulation, acne

Mascot: "Vinyl Es-trojan" + "Nora, Effin' drone"

> ➤ Combined oral contraceptive (COC) = birth control pill containing an estrogen + a progestin

> ➤ Ethinyl estradiol is a vinyl-covered Trojan horse – "Es-trojan" for estrogen

> ➤ "Nora, Effin' drone" – norethindrone, the progestin

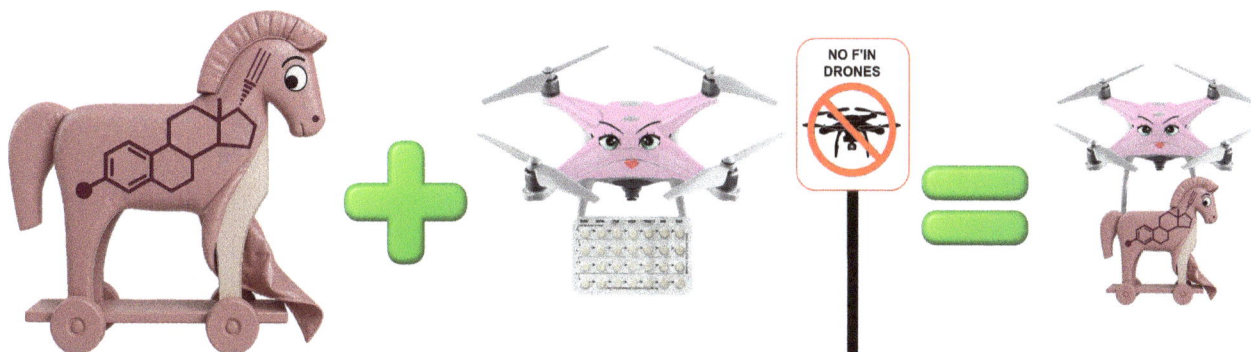

Alternate Mnemonics:

❖ "Ethinyl like vinyl" – EE is a synthetic estrogen

❖ "Ethinyl's in the pill pack", Estradiol (natural estrogen) is in patches and vaginal gels/creams/etc

❖ "LOESTRIN = low estrogen" – lower estrogen dose than older pills

❖ "MICROGESTIN = micro gestation prevention" (gestation = development of a fetus)

Drug Class: Hormonal contraceptive: Combined oral contraceptive (COC)

Similar Drugs: EE/Norgestimate (#99), EE/Levonorgestrel (#128), EE/Ethynodiol (#294)

Comparisons: Lower estrogen dose reduces nausea but increases breakthrough bleeding risk

High-Alert Risk: ⚠ ⚠ Increased risk of blood clots, especially in smokers >35

Major Side Effects: Nausea, breast tenderness, spotting

Narrow Therapeutic Index: No

Precautions: Avoid in women with clotting risk or estrogen-sensitive cancers; Must be taken at the same time every day

Routes: Oral

Easily Replaceable? Yes – other EE + progestin combos are comparable

Sample Test Questions:

Q: What is a serious risk of combined oral contraceptives?

A: Blood clots

Q: How should these pills be taken?

A: Daily, same time each day

Q: What estrogen is found in most combined oral contraceptives?

A: Ethinyl estradiol (EE)

#81 Lorazepam (ATIVAN)

lor-AZ-e-pam (AT-ih-van)

Common Uses: Anxiety, alcohol withdrawal, status epilepticus (to terminate a seizure)

Mascot: "Lorax's ATV"

➤ Commonly administered as an intramuscular injection in psychiatric hospitals

➤ In advanced CaferMed books, the troll-doll hair represents something related to drug-drug interactions (which are minimal with lorazepam)

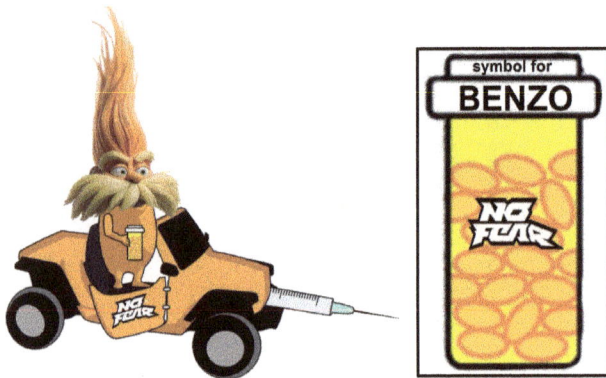

Alternate Mnemonics:

❖ "Pam = in the benzo fam" – -pam is a common benzodiazepine suffix

❖ "Ativan = acute anxiety vanisher"

Drug Class: Anxiolytic: Benzodiazepine

Similar Drugs: Clonazepam (#57), Diazepam (#169), Alprazolam (#41)

Comparisons: Intermediate-acting; preferred for liver impairment; fewer drug-drug interactions

Controlled Substance: ⚠ C-IV (Schedule IV) – like all benzos

High-Alert Risk: ⚠ ⚠ ⚠ Risk of respiratory depression, falls, and dependence

Major Side Effects: Drowsiness, confusion, dizziness, dependence

Look-Alike/Sound-Alike: Loxapine

Narrow Therapeutic Index: No

Precautions:

➤ Avoid with alcohol or opioids – risk of respiratory depression and death

➤ Avoid abrupt discontinuation due to potentially dangerous withdrawal with seizures

Routes: Oral, IV, IM

Easily Replaceable? Yes – dose conversions defined with other benzos

Also: Benzo withdrawal is nearly identical to alcohol withdrawal

Sample Test Questions:

Q: What is a key withdrawal risk when a benzodiazepine is abruptly stopped?

A: Seizures

#82 Quetiapine (SEROQUEL)

kweh-TYE-ah-peen (SAIR-oh-kwell)

Common Uses: Schizophrenia, bipolar disorder, depression (add-on), insomnia (off-label)

Mascot: "Sera, Quit typing!"

➤ Antipsychotics are represented by spooky mascots

➤ "'Sera, quit typing – it's time to sleep!'" – treatment for manic episodes

➤ **Polka dots on pink = alpha-1 blockade → orthostatic hypotension and fainting ("hit the floor")**

➤ H1 antihistamines may cause sedation and weight gain

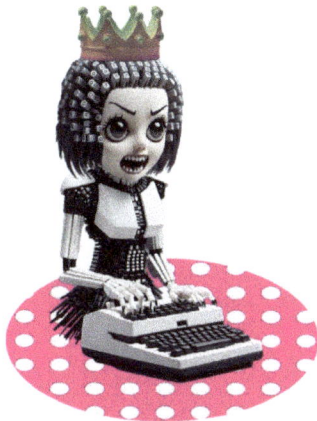

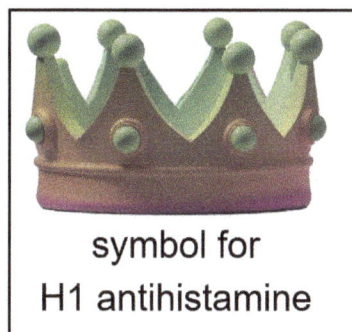

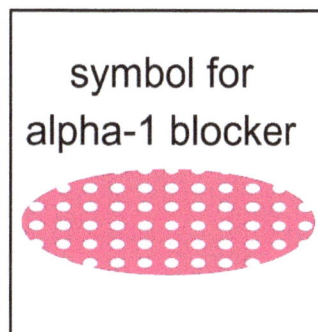

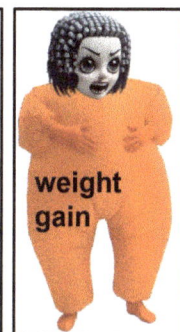

symbol for
H1 antihistamine

symbol for
alpha-1 blocker

weight gain

Alternate Mnemonics:

❖ "Quetiapine = quiets the mind"

❖ "Seroquel = serotonin + quelling" – blocks serotonin receptors (also dopamine receptors)

Drug Class: Antipsychotic: Atypical (2nd generation) antipsychotic – dopamine and serotonin receptor blocker

Similar Drugs: Aripiprazole (#106), Risperidone (#183), Olanzapine (#171)

Comparisons: More sedating; lower extrapyramidal side effects (EPS = muscle stiffness, restlessness, or shaking caused by antipsychotics); More weight gain than aripiprazole but less than olanzapine

Controlled Substance: ✅ Not controlled – all antipsychotics are non-controlled

High-Alert Risk: ⚠️ ⚠️ Risk of diabetes, sedation, and QT prolongation (cardiac conduction disturbance)

Major Side Effects: Weight gain, sedation, dry mouth, low blood pressure, fainting

Narrow Therapeutic Index: No

Precautions: Monitor weight, blood sugars, and lipids

Routes: Oral

Easily Replaceable? No – among antipsychotics, quetiapine has unique properties

Also: Extended release (XR) and immediate release (IR) forms are not interchangeable

Sample Test Questions:

Q: What class is quetiapine?

A: Atypical (2nd generation) antipsychotic

#83 Budesonide + Formoterol (SYMBICORT)

byoo-DESS-oh-nide; for-MOE-ter-ol (SIM-bih-cort)

Common Uses: Asthma, Chronic Obstructive Pulmonary Disease (COPD)

Mascot: "Air Bud" (PULMACORT) + "Formal air 'n' all" = "Buds, Formally"

➤ Don't confuse the golden retriever for a lab — Budesonide's the steroid; Formoterol's the LABA

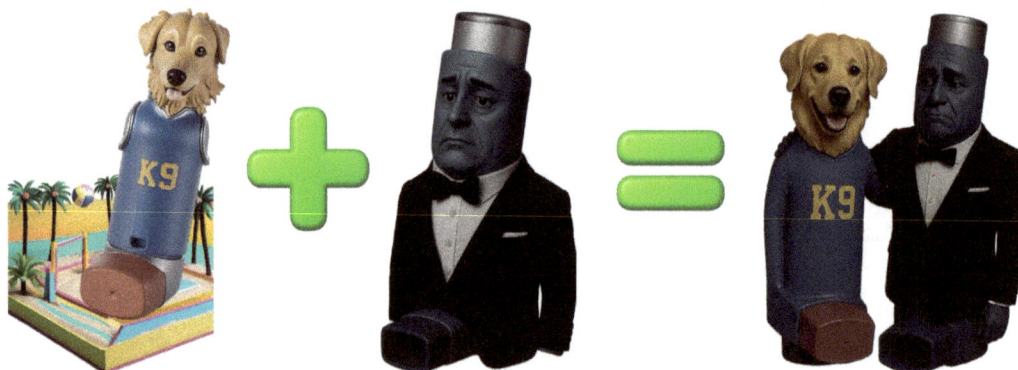

Alternate Mnemonics:

❖ "Symbicort = symbiotic corticosteroid (and LABA)"

Drug Class: Respiratory: Inhaled corticosteroid (ICS) + long-acting beta agonist (LABA)

Similar Drugs: Fluticasone/Salmeterol (#59), Fluticasone/Vilanterol (#145)

Comparisons: Formoterol has faster onset than salmeterol; may be used as rescue + controller

High-Alert Risk: ✅ Not high risk

Major Side Effects: Oral thrush, tremor, headache, cough

Look-Alike/Sound-Alike: Symbyax

Narrow Therapeutic Index: No

Precautions: Rinse mouth after use to prevent thrush (yeast infection of mouth or throat)

Routes: Inhalation

Easily Replaceable? Yes – other ICS + LABA combos are comparable

Also: In SMART protocols, formoterol allows use for rescue and maintenance

Sample Test Questions:

Q: What classes of medications are contained in Symbicort?

A: Inhaled corticosteroid (ICS) + long-acting beta agonist (LABA)

Q: Is budesonide or formoterol the corticosteroid?

A: Budesonide

Q: What is a side effect of budesonide-containing inhalers?

A: Thrush

Q: What class is formoterol?

A: Long-acting beta agonist (LABA)

Q: Is Symbicort used for quick relief?

A: Yes, it can be in SMART (Single Maintenance And Reliever Therapy) protocols

#84 Topiramate (TOPAMAX)

toe-PEER-a-mate (TOE-puh-max)

Common Uses: Epilepsy, migraine prevention, weight loss (off-label), psychiatric uses (off-label)

Mascot: "Top at max at Top of pyramid"

➤ Kidney throwing stones – can cause kidney stones

➤ The 'A' on the pyramid reminds you: topirAmate / topAmax – not "topirimate"

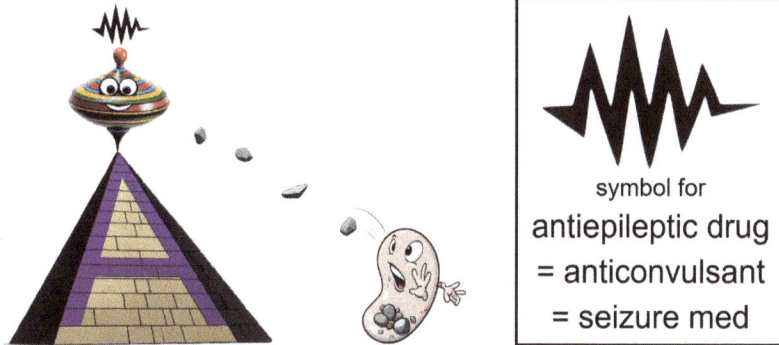

symbol for
**antiepileptic drug
= anticonvulsant
= seizure med**

Alternate Mnemonics:

❖ "Topamax = top off seizures + migraines"

❖ Has been nicknamed "Dopamax" or "Stupamax" for brain fog / word-finding difficulties > 200 mg/day

❖ "Topiramate = top irritant to memory" > 200 mg/day

Drug Class: Anticonvulsant: Sodium channel blocker

Similar Drugs: Valproate (#174), Lamotrigine (#58), Levetiracetam (#123)

Comparisons: Fewer side effects than valproate; Cognitive slowing is more common with topiramate than with lamotrigine or levetiracetam

Controlled Substance: ✅ Not controlled

High-Alert Risk: ⚠️ ⚠️ Risk of metabolic acidosis, cognitive impairment, kidney stones

Major Side Effects: Confusion, paresthesias, weight loss, kidney stones

Look-Alike/Sound-Alike: Toprol

Narrow Therapeutic Index: No

Precautions: Ensure adequate hydration to reduce stone risk

Routes: Oral

Easily Replaceable? No – topiramate has unique properties

Also: Approved for weight loss in combo with phentermine

Sample Test Questions:

Q: What side effect is common with topiramate above 200 mg / day?

A: Word-finding difficulty – "Dopamax"

Q: Why should patients hydrate while on topiramate?

A: To avoid kidney stones

#85 Warfarin (COUMADIN)

WAR-fuh-rin (KOO-muh-din, JAN-toe-ven)

Common Uses: Anticoagulant ("blood thinner") for prevention of stroke in atrial fibrillation (A-fib) or with prosthetic heart valves; Treatment and prevention of deep vein thrombosis (DVT) and pulmonary embolism (PE)

Mascot: "Warfare Comin' down"

> ➤ Warfarin blocks vitamin K from helping make clotting factors; Vitamin K is also the warfarin antidote

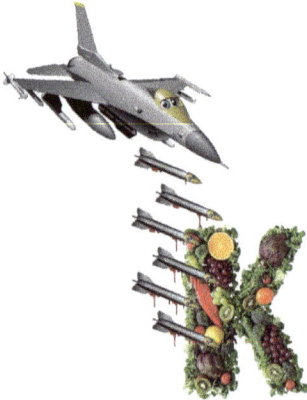

Alternate Mnemonics:

* ❖ "Coumadin = coagulation commander"
* ❖ "INR = I Need Regular-checks" – International Normalized Ratio (INR)
* ❖ "Rat poison with precision" – originally developed as a rodenticide

Drug Class: Anticoagulant: Vitamin K antagonist (blocker)

Similar Drugs: Apixaban (#27), Rivaroxaban (#90)

Comparisons: Warfarin requires monitoring; Warfarin has food and drug interactions

High-Alert Risk: ⚠ ⚠ ⚠ ⚠ High bleed risk; INR must be monitored

> ➤ INR (International Normalized Ratio) = time for blood to clot ≈ 1.0 for people not on warfarin
> ➤ Target INR is 2.0–3.0 for most indications, 2.5–3.5 for mechanical mitral valve

Major Side Effects: Bleeding, bruising, skin necrosis

> ➤ Purple toe syndrome – rare warfarin side effect when small cholesterol clots block toe vessels

Narrow Therapeutic Index: ⚠ ⚠ ⚠ ⚠ Yes

Precautions: Monitor INR closely, maintain consistent vitamin K intake

Routes: Oral

Easily Replaceable? No – the only appropriate oral anticoagulant with mechanical heart valves.

Also: Often bridged with heparin at first, since warfarin takes several days to work

Sample Test Questions:

Q: What lab value is monitored with warfarin?

A: INR (how long blood takes to clot)

Q: What's the antidote for warfarin?

A: Vitamin K

#86 Sitagliptin (JANUVIA)

SIT-a-glip-tin (JAN-you-vee-uh)

Common Uses: Type 2 diabetes

Mascot: "Sittin-gliptin, That's Januvia – Sittin' down would behoove ya'" (rhyme)

➤ Gliptins = the opposite of Lipton tea — unsweet, DPP-4–blocking teabags

➤ *Sitaglipton* on the album *Dipeptidyl Peptidase-4 Inhibitors* is available on YouTube, Spotify, etc

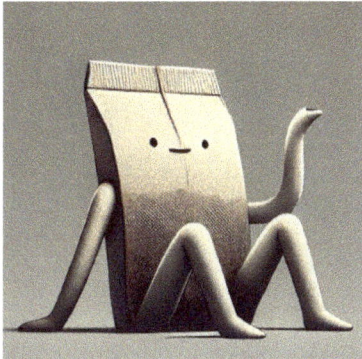

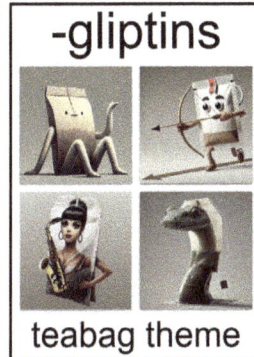

-gliptins

teabag theme

Alternate Mnemonics:

❖ "Sitagliptin = sits on DPP-4" – the enzyme gliptins inhibit

Drug Class: Antidiabetic: DPP-4 inhibitor

Similar Drugs: Linagliptin (not Top 300)

Comparisons: Weight neutral, low risk of hypoglycemia; Less effective than GLP-1 agonists

High-Alert Risk: ✅ Not high alert

Major Side Effects: Nasopharyngitis (inflammation of the nose / throat), headache, pancreatitis, joint pain

Look-Alike/Sound-Alike: Janumet

Narrow Therapeutic Index: No

Precautions: Monitor for signs of pancreatitis, especially abdominal pain

Routes: Oral

Easily Replaceable? Yes – other DPP-4 inhibitors (-gliptins) are comparable

Also: Often combined with metformin in the combo product Janumet

Sample Test Questions:

Q: What enzyme does sitagliptin inhibit?

A: DPP-4

Q: What's the result of DPP-4 inhibition?

A: Prolonged incretin activity (e.g., GLP-1)

Q: What's a rare but serious side effect?

A: Pancreatitis

Q: Is sitagliptin associated with weight gain or loss?

A: Neither – weight neutral

#87 Amitriptyline (ELAVIL)

a-mee-TRIP-ti-leen (ELL-uh-vil)

Common Uses: Depression, headache prevention, neuropathic pain, insomnia

Mascot: "Amy tripping off the Elevator"

➤ Among antidepressant medications, amitriptyline has maximum side effects

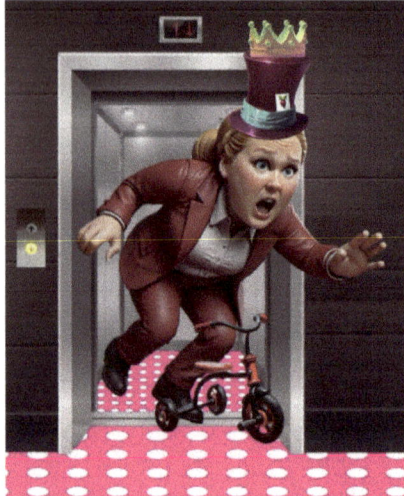

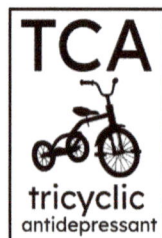

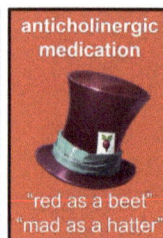

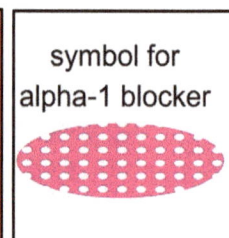

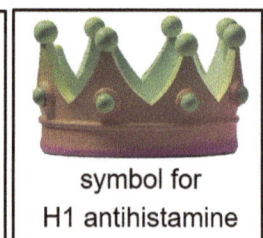

TCA — tricyclic antidepressant

anticholinergic medication — "red as a beet" "mad as a hatter"

symbol for alpha-1 blocker

symbol for H1 antihistamine

Alternate Mnemonics:

❖ "Triptyline = triple threat"

  ➤ Anticholinergic – dry mouth, constipation, urinary retention, confusion, ↓ sweating ("red as a beet")

  ➤ Antihistamine – sedation, most weight gain of any antidepressant

  ➤ Alpha blocker – low blood pressure when standing (orthostatic hypotension) → risk of fainting

❖ "Elavil elevates mood" – antidepressant

Drug Class: Antidepressant: Tricyclic Antidepressant (TCA)

Similar TCAs: Nortriptyline (#191), Doxepin (#218)

Comparisons: More side effects than nortriptyline

Controlled Substance: ✅ Not controlled

High-Alert Risk: ⚠️⚠️⚠️ Overdose may cause fatal arrhythmias; High fall risk in older adults

Major Side Effects: Sedation, dry mouth, constipation, dizziness, weight gain

Look-Alike/Sound-Alike: Amantadine, Amoxapine

Narrow Therapeutic Index: ⚠️ Yes – TCAs may cause fatal cardiac arrhythmias at high dose

Precautions: Avoid in elderly due to anticholinergic burden

Routes: Oral

Easily Replaceable? Yes – several TCAs have better tolerability than amitriptyline

Sample Test Questions:

Q: Why is amitriptyline dangerous in overdose?

A: It can cause fatal heart arrhythmias

#88 Fenofibrate (TRICOR)

FEN-oh-fye-brate (TRY-core)
Common Uses: To decrease high triglycerides
Mascot: "Feno's fibrous Tricorne / Tri-cord"

➤ He's wearing a tricorn hat

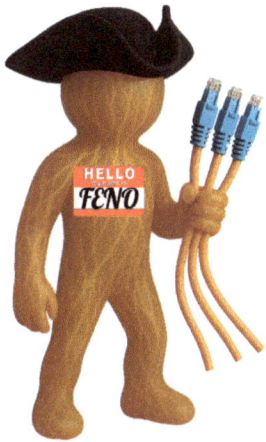

Alternate Mnemonics:

❖ "Fibrates fights fat"

❖ "Tricor = triglyceride corrector"

❖ "TRICOR lowers TRIglycerides to help CORonary artery disease"

❖ "Fenofibrate = fatty foam fixer"

Drug Class: Lipid-lowering: Fibric acid derivative
Similar Drugs: Gemfibrozil (#231)
Comparisons: Better at lowering triglycerides and fewer drug interactions than gemfibrozil
High-Alert Risk: ✅ Not high alert
Major Side Effects: GI upset, muscle pain (especially with statins), elevated liver enzymes, gallstones
Narrow Therapeutic Index: No
Precautions: Monitor liver enzymes; Use caution in kidney impairment
Routes: Oral
Easily Replaceable? Yes – gemfibrozil is comparable

Sample Test Questions:
Q: What is fenofibrate used for?
A: High triglycerides
Q: Is fenofibrate a statin?
A: No – it's a fibrate
Q: What side effect can occur when fenofibrate is combined with a statin?
A: Muscle toxicity (myopathy)

#89 Naproxen (ALEVE)

NAH-prox-en (uh-LEEV, NAP-ro-sin)
Common Uses: NSAID for pain, arthritis
Mascot: "Nap-rocks (on) A levee"

➤ "nap-rocks" - rocks to nap on

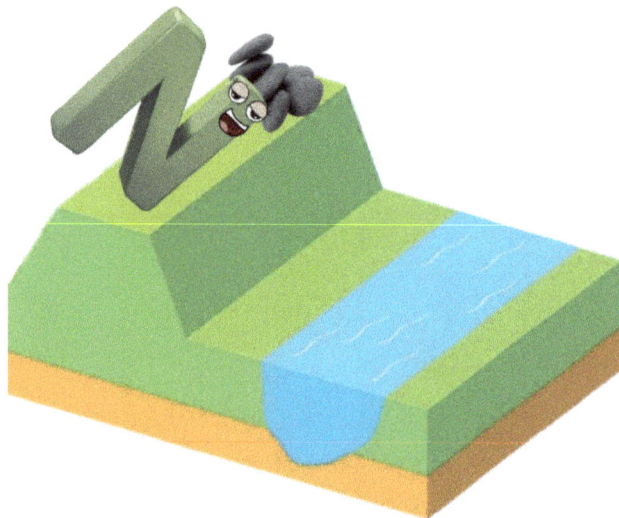

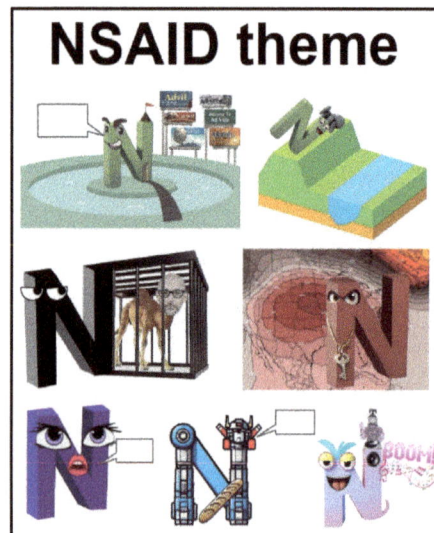

NSAID theme

Alternate Mnemonics:

❖ "Aleve = Allieve pain"

❖ "NSAID with longer action"

❖ "N-Prox = NSAID with proximity to pain relief"

Drug Class: Anti-inflammatory: NSAID (nonselective COX inhibitor)
Similar Drugs: Ibuprofen (#33), Diclofenac (#51), Meloxicam (#29)
Comparisons: Longer-acting than ibuprofen
Controlled Substance: ✅ Not controlled – no NSAIDs are controlled
High-Alert Risk: ⚠️ ⚠️ GI bleed, kidney injury, cardiovascular risk
Major Side Effects: GI upset, stomach ulcers, increased blood pressure, renal toxicity
Look-Alike/Sound-Alike: Nexium
Narrow Therapeutic Index: No
Precautions: Avoid in kidney disease or recent cardiac events: Take with food to reduce GI upset
Routes: Oral
Easily Replaceable? Yes – other NSAIDs are comparable

Sample Test Questions:
Q: Is naproxen selective for COX-2?
A: No – it blocks both COX-1 and COX-2
Q: What organ can be affected by chronic use of NSAIDs?
A: Kidneys

#90 Rivaroxaban (XARELTO)

RIV-a-ROX-a-ban (zah-RELL-toh)

Common Uses: Anticoagulant ("blood thinner") for prevention of stroke in atrial fibrillation (A-fib), Treatment and prevention of deep vein thrombosis (DVT) and pulmonary embolism (PE)

Mascot: "(By) Czar Realtor's (decree): River rocks are banned"

➤ Xa-ban mascots wear a BANdana and are "banned" (as a mnemonic, not literally)

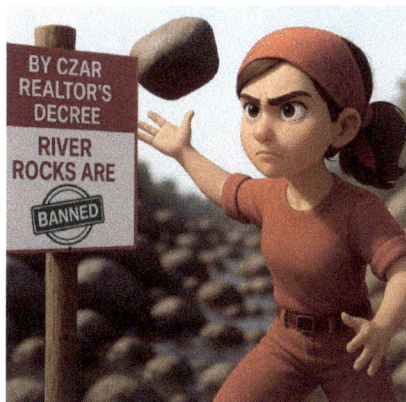

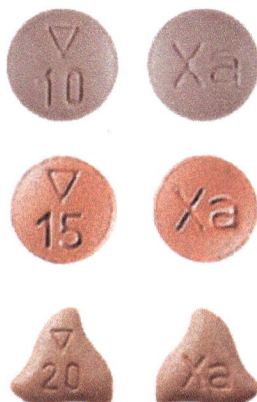

Alternate Mnemonics:

❖ "Rivaro-Xa-ban rocks factor Xa"

❖ *Rivaroxaban* song available on YouTube, Spotify, etc

Drug Class: Anticoagulant: Direct Factor Xa inhibitor (DOAC)

Similar Drugs: Apixaban (#27), Warfarin (#85)

Comparisons: Shorter half-life, no INR monitoring, fewer food interactions than warfarin

➤ INR (International Normalized Ratio) measures how long blood takes to clot; normal INR is ~1.0

High-Alert Risk: ⚠ ⚠ ⚠ High bleed risk, especially with kidney impairment or age >75

Major Side Effects: Bleeding, bruising, anemia, nausea

Look-Alike/Sound-Alike: Xalatan

Narrow Therapeutic Index: No

Precautions: Dose adjustment in kidney impairment

Routes: Oral

Easily Replaceable? Yes – other DOACs are comparable

Also: Can be reversed with andexanet alfa (which also has Xa in the name)

Sample Test Questions:

Q: What factor does rivaroxaban inhibit?

A: Factor Xa (it's in the name)

Q: What's a major risk with Xarelto?

A: Bleeding

Q: Does it require INR monitoring like warfarin?

A: No

#91 Pregabalin (LYRICA)

pree-GAB-a-lin (LEER-ih-kuh)

Common Uses: Neuropathy (nerve pain), fibromyalgia, seizures, anxiety

Mascot: "Preg gobblin' Lyrics"

➤ She's pregnant – see the turkey embryo? (incidentally, it should be avoided in pregnancy unless essential)

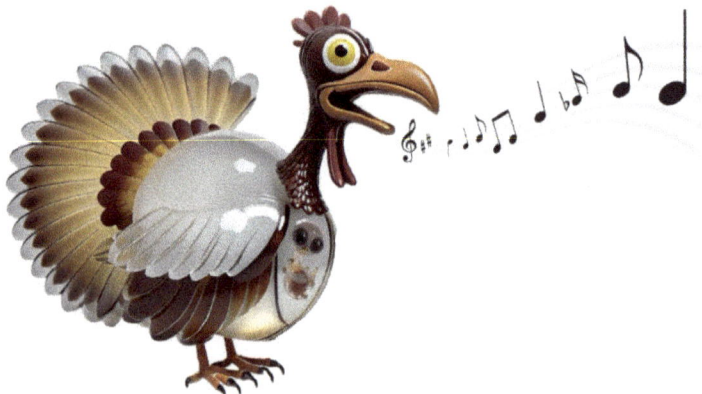

Alternate Mnemonics:

❖ Pre-GABA-lin resembles GABA, a calming neurotransmitter

❖ "Lyrica lyrics" of *Pregabalin* song available on YouTube, Spotify, etc – useful for memorizing dosing

Drug Class: Antiepileptic (antiseizure medication): gabapentinoid

Similar Drugs: Gabapentin (#10)

Comparisons: Faster onset and more predictable absorption than gabapentin; Gabapentin is not a federally controlled substance; Edema (leg swelling) is more common with pregabalin

Controlled Substance: ⚠ C-V = the least restrictive schedule

➤ Mild abuse potential – causes euphoria in some

High-Alert Risk: ⚠ CNS depression (sedation), misuse risk, falls in elderly

Major Side Effects: Dizziness, somnolence, edema, weight gain

Look-Alike/Sound-Alike: Lamisil

Narrow Therapeutic Index: No

Precautions: Taper to avoid withdrawal; Caution in kidney impairment

Routes: Oral

Easily Replaceable? Yes – similar to gabapentin

Sample Test Questions:

Q: Is pregabalin a controlled substance?

A: Yes – C-V

Q: What's pregabalin used for?

A: Neuropathic pain, seizures, fibromyalgia

#92 Paroxetine (PAXIL)

PAIR-ox-uh-teen (PACKS-ill)

Common Uses: Depression, anxiety

Mascot: "Pear rocks a teen (Paxil Rose)"

➤ Anticholinergic effects aren't strong enough to earn the paroxetine mascot a mad-hatter hat (like amitriptyline), but Paxil is the only SSRI with anticholinergic effects — symbolized by crimson roses

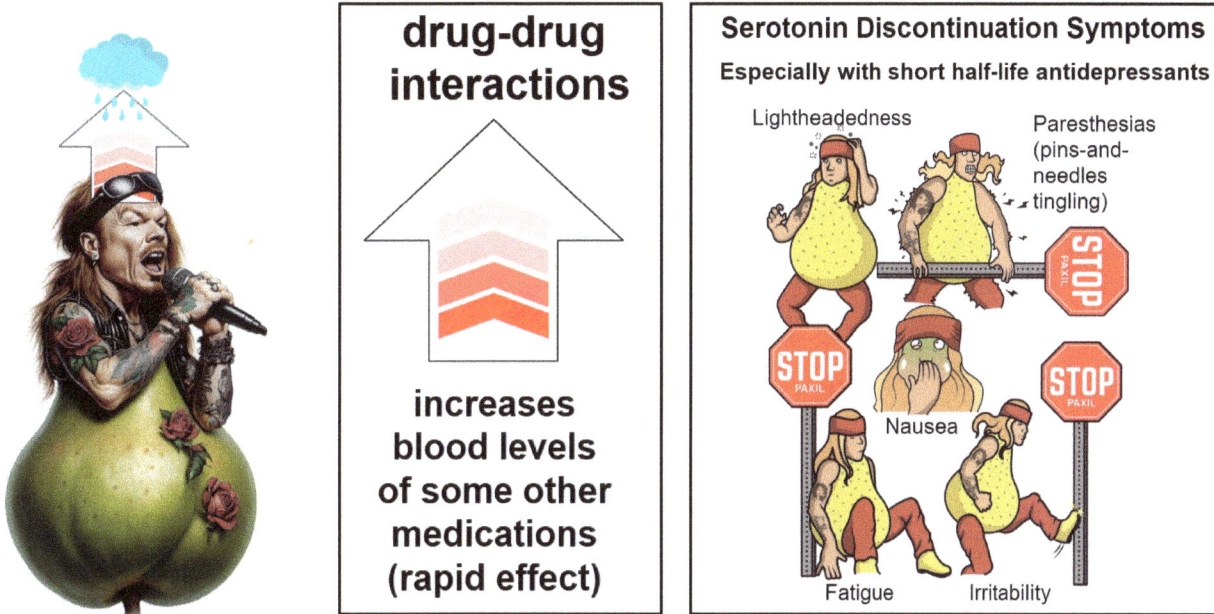

drug-drug interactions

increases blood levels of some other medications (rapid effect)

Serotonin Discontinuation Symptoms

Especially with short half-life antidepressants

Lightheadedness

Paresthesias (pins-and-needles tingling)

STOP PAXIL

STOP PAXIL

STOP PAXIL

Nausea

Fatigue   Irritability

Alternate Mnemonics:

❖ "Paxil packs it in" – constipation

Drug Class: Antidepressant: SSRI (Selective Serotonin Reuptake Inhibitor)

Similar Drugs: Sertraline (#11), Fluoxetine (#22), Citalopram (#40), Escitalopram (#15)

Comparisons: The only anticholinergic SSRI; Short half-life → faster/worse withdrawal; Most sexual side effects among SSRIs; 2nd most interactions (after fluoxetine); The least safe SSRI during pregnancy

Controlled Substance: ✅ Not controlled

High-Alert Risk: ⚠ Suicidal thoughts in patients younger than 25 – warning applicable to all antidepressants; Discontinuation syndrome (withdrawal – uncomfortable but not physically dangerous)

Major Side Effects: Weight gain, sexual dysfunction, dry mouth, withdrawal

Look-Alike/Sound-Alike: Plavix

Narrow Therapeutic Index: No

Precautions: Taper very slowly; Avoid in pregnancy

Easily Replaceable? Partially – SSRIs are similar, but psychiatric medications often require trial and error

Sample Test Questions:

Q: Why is paroxetine harder to stop than other SSRIs?

A: Short half-life → faster/more severe withdrawal

#93 Celecoxib (CELEBREX)

SELL-eh-cox-ib (SELL-eh-brex)
Common Uses: Pain, arthritis
Mascot: "2 Celebrating Cocks"
➤ Selective COX-2 inhibitor

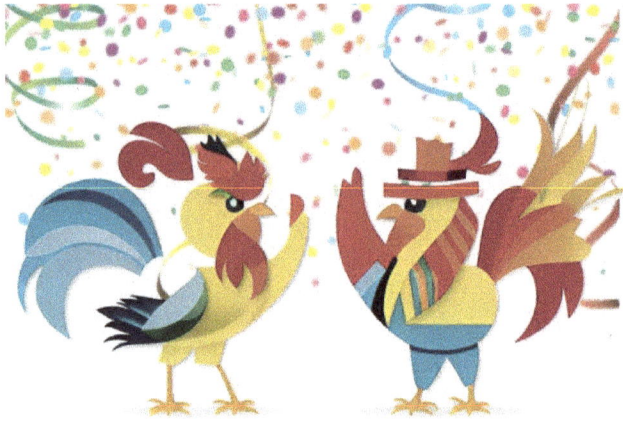

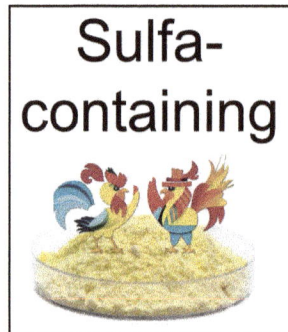

Sulfa-containing

Alternate Mnemonics:

❖ "Celebrate fewer ulcers"

❖ *Celecoxib* song available on YouTube, Spotify, etc

Drug Class: Nonsteroidal Anti-inflammatory Drug (NSAID): COX-2 selective
Similar Drugs: Meloxicam (#29) – COX-2 preferring but still inhibits COX-1
Comparisons: Lower GI risk than non-selective NSAIDs
Controlled Substance: ✅ Not controlled
High-Alert Risk: ⚠ Increased heart attack / stroke risk; renal injury
Major Side Effects: Hypertension, edema, GI discomfort
Look-Alike/Sound-Alike: Celexa
Narrow Therapeutic Index: No
Precautions: Use lowest effective dose
Routes: Oral
Easily Replaceable? Yes – other NSAIDs are comparable but higher GI risk
Also: Contains sulfa group – caution with allergy, although cross-reactivity with sulfa antibiotics is low

Sample Test Questions:
Q: What's a serious cardiovascular risk of celecoxib?
A: Increased risk of heart attack and stroke
Q: Is celecoxib safer on the stomach?
A: Yes – less GI toxicity
Q: Can celecoxib be used in sulfa-allergic patients?
A: Caution – it contains a sulfa group

#94 Tizanidine (ZANAFLEX)

tih-ZAN-ih-deen (ZAN-uh-flex)
Common Uses: Muscle spasm, spasticity
Mascot: "Zany flex in a Tizzy"

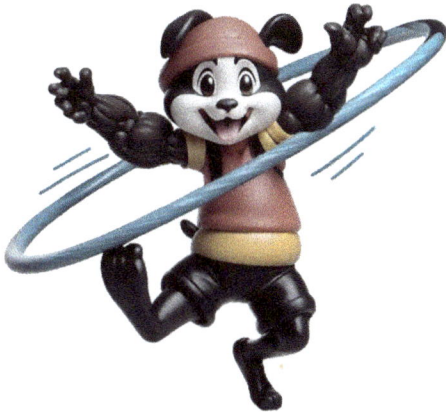

Alternate Mnemonics:
  ❖ "Tizanidine = ties up spasms"
Drug Class: Muscle relaxant: Central alpha-2 adrenergic agonist
  ➤ Activates alpha-2 receptors in the brain, which are a type of receptor for norepinephrine
Similar Drugs (different mechanisms): Cyclobenzaprine (#45), Baclofen (#104), Methocarbamol (#126)
Comparisons: More sedating than baclofen, shorter-acting
  ➤ Clonidine (#71) and Guanfacine (#275) are blood pressure-lowering medications that work as central alpha-2 agonists
Controlled Substance: ✅ Not controlled
High-Alert Risk: ⚠️ Sedation, hypotension (low blood pressure)
Major Side Effects: Drowsiness, dry mouth, hypotension, dizziness
Look-Alike/Sound-Alike: Zyrtec, Xanax
Narrow Therapeutic Index: No
Precautions: Avoid combining with alcohol or other sedating medications
Routes: Oral
Easily Replaceable? Yes – other muscle relaxants are comparable
Also: Take tizanidine with or without food — food increases absorption, so stay consistent

Sample Test Questions:
Q: What's a common side effect of tizanidine?
A: Sedation
Q: Can tizanidine lower blood pressure?
A: Yes – hypotension is common
Q: Should it be taken with food?
A: Be consistent – food increases absorption (it's stronger when taken with food)

#95 Sumatriptan (IMITREX)

SOO-mah-trip-tan (IM-ih-trex)
Common Uses: Acute migraine headaches
Mascot: "Sumo tripped In my tracks"

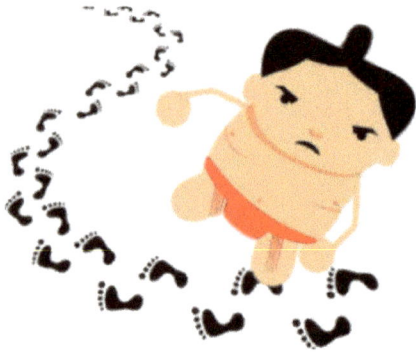

Alternate Mnemonics:

❖ "Suma trips up migraines fast"

❖ "I'm attacked? Trex it!"

Drug Class: Anti-migraine: serotonin receptor agonist (triptan)

➤ Stimulates serotonin (5-HT1B/1D) receptors to narrow blood vessels

Similar Drugs: Rizatriptan (#190)

Comparisons: Shorter-acting than others; nasal and injectable forms available

Controlled Substance: ✅ Not controlled

High-Alert Risk: ⚠️ ⚠️ Vasoconstriction – avoid in coronary artery disease, uncontrolled hypertension

Major Side Effects: Tingling, flushing, chest pressure, dizziness

Narrow Therapeutic Index: No

Precautions: Avoid within 24 hours of other triptans or ergotamines (older migraine drug that narrows blood vessels)

Routes: Oral, subcutaneous (SubQ), nasal

Easily Replaceable? Yes – other triptans are comparable

Also: Best taken at migraine onset for full effect

Sample Test Questions:

Q: What class of drug is sumatriptan?

A: Triptan (serotonin receptor agonist)

Q: What does sumatriptan do to blood vessels?

A: Narrows (constricts) them

Q: What is a serious side effect to watch for with sumatriptan?

A: Chest pain or tightness

Q: When should sumatriptan be taken?

A: At the first sign of migraine

#96 Amoxicillin + Clavulanate (AUGMENTIN)

uh-MOX-ih-sill-in; KLAV-yoo-luh-nayt (AWG-men-tin)

Common Uses: Antibiotic for sinus infections, ear infections, skin infections, pneumonia

Mascot: "Augmented Moxie" = "A Moxie ceiling" (Amoxicillin #26) + "Clavicle Annie" (Clavulanate)

➤ Both amoxicillin and clavulanate have a beta-lactam ring

◇ Amoxicillin is a beta-lactam antibiotic (a penicillin).

◇ Clavulanate is a beta-lactamase inhibitor that has little antibiotic activity on its own

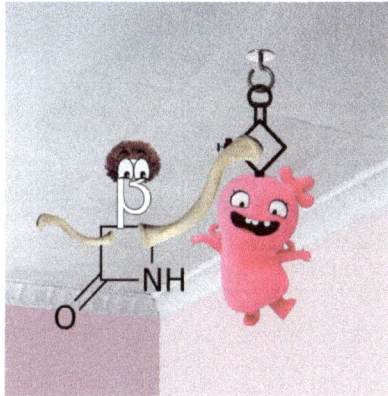

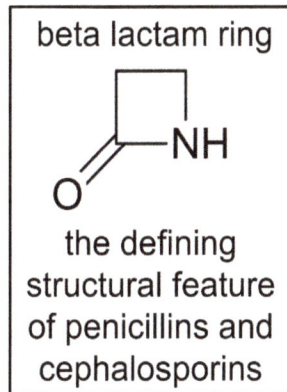

beta lactam ring

the defining structural feature of penicillins and cephalosporins

Alternate Mnemonics:

❖ "Augment = amoxicillin + reinforcement"

Drug Class: Antibiotic: β-lactam (amoxicillin) + β-lactamase inhibitor (clavulanate)

➤ Clavulanate blocks resistant bacteria from destroying amoxicillin's beta-lactam ring

Similar Drugs: Amoxicillin (#26), Cefuroxime (#283)

Comparisons: Covers more resistant organisms than amoxicillin alone

High-Alert Risk: ⚠ Allergic reaction, possible liver problems

Major Side Effects: Diarrhea, GI upset, rash, yeast infections

Look-Alike/Sound-Alike: Ampicillin, Azithromycin

Narrow Therapeutic Index: No

Precautions: Take with food to reduce GI upset; Watch for signs of allergy

Routes: Oral

Easily Replaceable? Yes – other penicillin combos or cephalosporins may substitute

Sample Test Questions:

Q: Why is amoxicillin often prescribed with clavulanate?

A. Clavulanate blocks bacteria from destroying amoxicillin's beta-lactam ring

Q: Should Augmentin be taken with food?

A: Yes – reduces GI upset

Q: What class of antibiotic is amoxicillin?

A: β-lactam antibiotic

#97 Olmesartan (BENICAR)

OLE-meh-sar-tan (BEN-ih-car)

Common Uses: Hypertension, kidney protection in diabetes

Mascot: "Be nicer, Omelette Sa(r)tan!"

➤ Olmesartan, but not other ARBs, is linked to sprue-like enteropathy (severe GI inflammation with diarrhea) → not very nice!

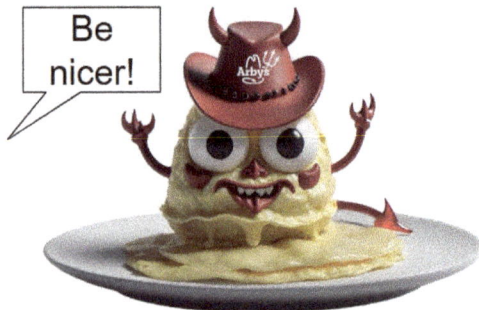

Be nicer!

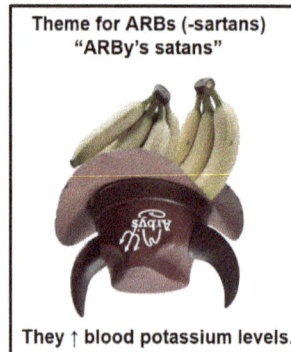

Theme for ARBs (-sartans)
"ARBy's satans"

They ↑ blood potassium levels.

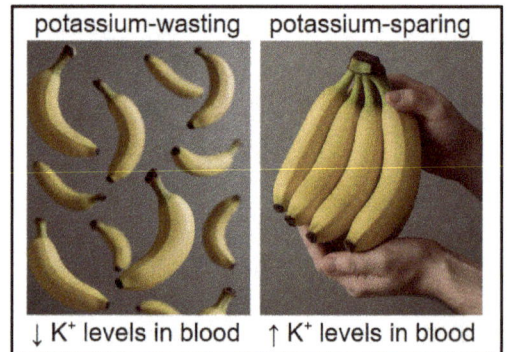

potassium-wasting   potassium-sparing

↓ K⁺ levels in blood   ↑ K⁺ levels in blood

Alternate Mnemonics:

❖ "Benicar = benefits the cardiovascular system"

❖ "Sartan = stops angiotensin II"

Drug Class: Angiotensin II Receptor Blocker (ARB)

Similar Drugs: Losartan (#8), Valsartan (#117)

Comparisons: Lower risk of cough or angioedema (severe swelling) than ACE inhibitors

High-Alert Risk: ⚠ Hyperkalemia (high potassium in blood), fetal toxicity

Major Side Effects: Dizziness, fatigue, hyperkalemia, kidney effects

Look-Alike/Sound-Alike: Benefiber, Benadryl

Narrow Therapeutic Index: No

Precautions: Avoid in pregnancy; Monitor potassium and kidney function

Routes: Oral

Easily Replaceable? Yes – other ARBs are comparable

Also: Rare but serious: sprue-like enteropathy with chronic diarrhea

Sample Test Questions:

Q: What class is olmesartan?

A: Angiotensin II Receptor Blocker (ARB)

Q: What serious risk does olmesartan pose in pregnancy?

A: Birth defects – applicable to all ACE inhibitors and ARBs

Q: Does olmesartan cause coughing?

A: No – unlike ACE inhibitors

Q: What labs should be monitored with olmesartan?

A: Potassium and kidney function

#98 Acetaminophen + Oxycodone (PERCOCET)

uh-SEE-tuh-MIN-uh-fen; OX-ee-KOH-dohn (PER-koh-set)

Common Uses: Moderate to severe pain

Mascot: "Perky Ox coding" for oxycodone

➤ See #114 for Acetaminophen mascot info

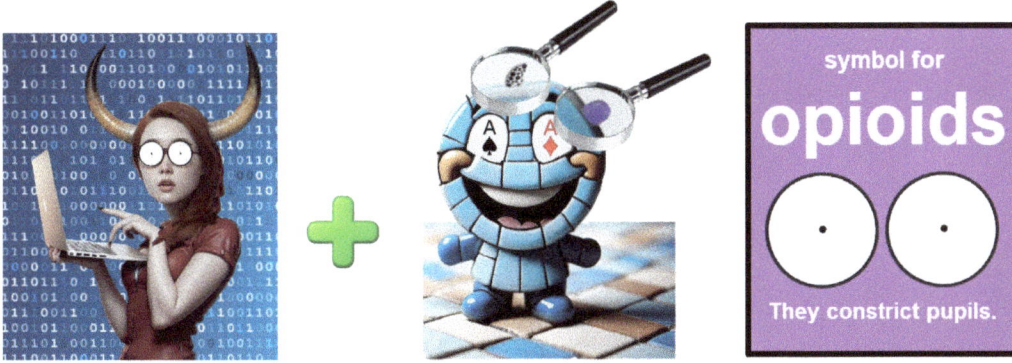

symbol for
opioids
They constrict pupils.

Alternate Mnemonics:

❖ "Percocet is the one with perks" – oxycodone is stronger and more requested than hydrocodone

Drug Class: Analgesic: Opioid + non-opioid combination

Similar Drugs: Acetaminophen (#114); Hydrocodone (#23), Tramadol (#55)

Comparisons: Oxycodone stronger than hydrocodone; higher abuse potential

Controlled Substance: ⚠ ⚠ ⚠ C-II

➤ High risk for abuse, dependence, overdose

High-Alert Risk: ⚠ ⚠ ⚠ ⚠

➤ Fatal overdose risk due to respiratory depression with oxycodone

➤ Liver toxicity from acetaminophen

Major Side Effects: Constipation, drowsiness, nausea, addiction

Look-Alike/Sound-Alike: Percocet vs. Percodan

Narrow Therapeutic Index: ⚠ Yes

Precautions: Avoid other sources of acetaminophen; Taper gradually if used long term to avoid opioid withdrawal

Routes: Oral

Easily Replaceable? Yes – other pain medications may substitute depending on severity

Sample Test Questions:

Q: What's the controlled status of Percocet?

A: C-II (Schedule II)

Q: What are the major safety risks of Percocet?

A: Respiratory depression and liver toxicity

Q: Is it safe to combine with other Tylenol products?

A: No – risk of liver damage

#99 Ethinyl Estradiol + Norgestimate (ORTHO TRI-CYCLEN)

ETH-in-il ES-truh-dye-ol; NOR-jes-ti-mayt (OR-tho try SYE-klen)
Common Uses: Contraception, acne, cycle regulation
Mascot: "Es-trojan" + "North estimator"

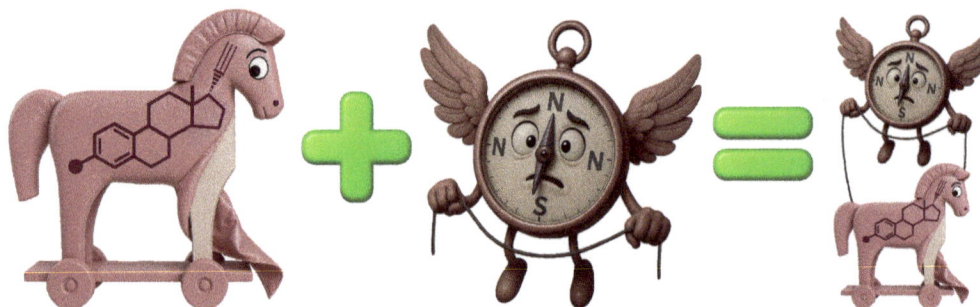

Alternate Mnemonics:

❖ "Ortho Tri = 3-phase timing" – Triphasic = hormone dose changes 3 times per cycle"

❖ "Norgest = next gen progestin"

Drug Class: Combined (estrogen + progestin) oral contraceptive (COC)
Similar Drugs: Ethinyl Estradiol (EE) + Norethindrone (#80), Drospirenone combos (#142, #285)
Comparisons: Triphasic – varies hormone levels across cycle
Controlled Substance: ✅ Not controlled
High-Alert Risk: ⚠️ ⚠️ Blood clot risk, especially in smokers >35
Major Side Effects: Nausea, spotting, headache, breast tenderness
Look-Alike/Sound-Alike: Tri-Sprintec
Narrow Therapeutic Index: No
Precautions: Take at same time daily
Routes: Oral
Easily Replaceable? Yes – other combination OCPs are comparable

Sample Test Questions:
Q: What's the main use of Ortho Tri-Cyclen?
A: Birth control
Q: What's a major safety risk?
A: Blood clots, especially in smokers > age 35
Q: How many phases are in this pill?
A: Three (triphasic)
Q: What two hormone types are in it?
A: Estrogen and progestin
Q: What's a common non-contraceptive reason to prescribe Ortho Tri-Cyclen?
A: Acne treatment or cycle regulation

#100 Diltiazem (CARDIZEM)

DIL-tye-a-zem (KAR-dih-zem)
Common Uses: Hypertension, angina (cardiac chest pain), atrial fibrillation (irregular heart rhythm)
Mascot: "Dill ties a Cardigan"

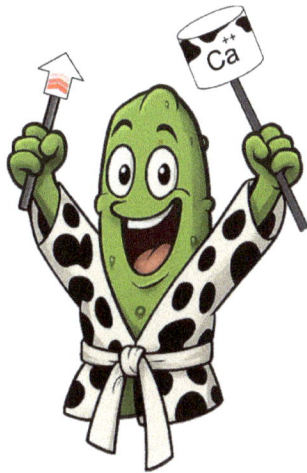

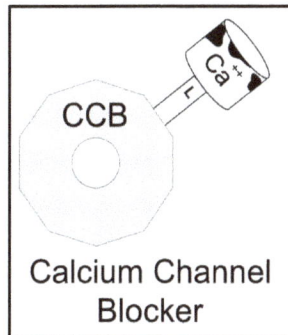

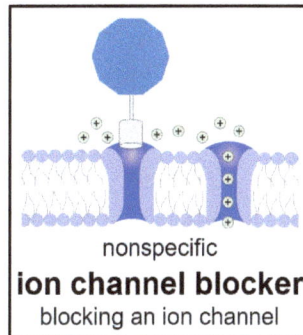

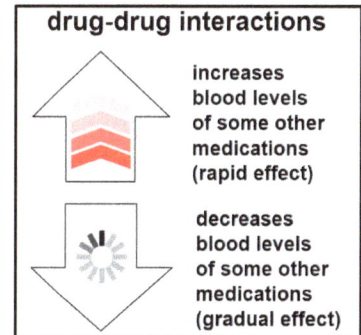

Calcium Channel Blocker

nonspecific
ion channel blocker
blocking an ion channel

drug-drug interactions

increases blood levels of some other medications (rapid effect)

decreases blood levels of some other medications (gradual effect)

Alternate Mnemonics:

❖ *Calcium Channel Blockers* song available on YouTube, Spotify, etc

Drug Class: Calcium channel blocker (CCB): non-dihydropyridine
Similar Drugs: Verapamil (#188)
Comparisons: Like verapamil (the other non-dihydropyridine CCB), diltiazem reduces blood pressure (BP) and slows conduction in the heart; Dihydropyridine CCBs like Amlodipine (#5) and Nifedipine (#155) reduce BP but do not slow conduction

➤ Less constipation than verapamil

High-Alert Risk: ⚠️ ⚠️ Hypotension, Bradycardia (slow heart rate), AV block = delayed or blocked signal between atria and ventricles
Major Side Effects: Edema, fatigue, constipation, dizziness
Look-Alike/Sound-Alike: Diazepam, Cardene
Narrow Therapeutic Index: No
Precautions: Do not use with beta-blockers (propranolol, metoprolol) unless heart rate and BP monitored
Routes: Oral, IV
Easily Replaceable? Yes – though among CCBs only verapamil and diltiazem provide heart rhythm control

Sample Test Questions:
Q: What kind of calcium blocker is diltiazem?
A: Non-dihydropyridine (along with verapamil)
Q: What are diltiazem and verapamil used for besides blood pressure?
A: Atrial fibrillation rate control and angina

Where are #101 – #113?

#114 Acetaminophen (TYLENOL) is provided to explain:

❖ #23 Hydrocodone/Acetaminophen (VICODIN, NORCO)

❖ #98 Acetaminophen + Oxycodone (PERCOCET)

The collection of medication mascots is expanding. In higher-level CaferMed books, mascots evolve into data-driven interaction avatars designed for memorization of specific drug-drug interactions.

Visit cafermed.com/subscribe for medications beyond #100.

#114 Acetaminophen (Paracetamol, APAP, TYLENOL)

Common Uses: Pain and fever

Mascot: "I see the mini fin, a Pair a' aces, A papule, Tile 'n' all"

❖ "I see the mini fin" for acetaminophen

❖ "Pair a' aces" = paracetamol (common name outside U.S.)

❖ "A papule" for APAP = N-acetyl-para-aminophenol – chemical name used in combination products such as Hydrocodone/APAP and Oxycodone/APAP

❖ "Tile n' all" for Tylenol

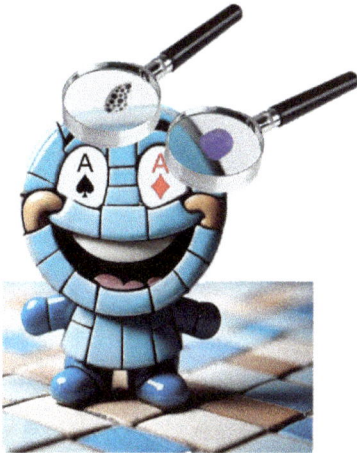

Drug Class: Analgesic / Antipyretic (fever reducer) — not an opioid or NSAID

Similar Drugs: None

Comparisons: Relieves pain and fever — but not inflammation; Safer on the stomach than NSAIDs; Does not thin blood like aspirin

High-Alert Risk: ⚠ ⚠ ⚠ Severe liver damage, especially if over 4,000 mg/day; Watch for hidden APAP in combo meds; The 4,000 mg/day limit applies to acetaminophen from all sources

Major Side Effects: Liver damage (high doses), rash (rare)

Look-Alike/Sound-Alike: Acetazolamide

Narrow Therapeutic Index: No — but serious liver damage in overdose

Precautions: Caution in liver disease; Avoid alcohol (adds liver strain); Check all meds for APAP content

Routes: Oral (tabs, caps, liquid), Rectal, IV

Easily Replaceable? Partially — Acetaminophen is unique but other pain medications are available

Also: Safe in pregnancy when used as directed

Sample Test Questions:

Q: What is the main risk of acetaminophen over 4,000 mg/day?

A: Serious liver damage

Q: What does APAP stand for on medication labels?

A: Acetaminophen (short for its chemical name)

Q: Why is it important to check all meds for APAP?

A To avoid accidental acetaminophen overdose from multiple sources

Drug Prefixes Guide

Prefix	Drug Class	Examples	Mnemonic / Background
ar-	The right-handed half of what used to be a 50/50 mix	Armodafinil Arformoterol Arketamine	❖ "ar-" = (R) configuration (right-handed) ➤ opposite of "es-" = (S) ❖ Usually a cleaner version of an older drug that was a 50:50 mix of (R)- and (S)-
calc-	Vitamin D analogs ➤ Calcium-related meds	Calcitriol Calcitonin	❖ "CALC = CALCium control"
cef- / ceph-	Cephalosporin antibiotics	Cephalexin Cefdinir	❖ "Ceph = cephalopod tentacles grabbing bacteria"
cyclo-	Molecule that contains one or more rings	Cyclophosphamide Cyclobenzaprine	❖ "CYCLO = Cyclic"
des-	A simplified version with one methyl group ($-CH_3$) removed	Desvenlafaxine Desipramine Desloratadine	❖ "des-" = desmethylated ❖ Example: desipramine = imipramine minus CH_3
dex-	The version that rotates light to the right	Dextroamphetamine Dexmethylphenidate Dextromethorphan Dexlansoprazole Dexmedetomidine Dexchlorphenir-amine	❖ DEX- for dextrous (right-handed) ➤ opposite of LEVO- ❖ Usually a cleaner version of an older drug that was a 50/50 mix ❖ Not necessarily a right-handed (R)-enantiomer – in some instances the (L)-enantiomer rotates light to the right
epo-	Erythropoiesis-stimulating agents ➤ ↑ red blood cells (RBCs) to treat anemia	Epoetin Darbepoetin	❖ "EPO = ErythroPOiesis booster" ❖ e-ryth-ro-poi-e-sis = production of erythrocytes (RBCs)

es-	The left-handed half of what used to be a 50/50 mix	Escitalopram Esomeprazole Esketamine Eszopiclone	❖ "Es-" for (S) = "sinister" (left-handed) ➤ opposite of "ar-" = (R) ❖ Usually a cleaner version of an older drug that was a 50:50 mix of (R)- and (S)-
gli- / gly-	Sulfonylureas ➤ diabetes meds	Glipizide Glyburide	❖ -gly for glycemic = related to glucose
hydroxy-	Has an OH (hydroxyl) group	Hydroxychloroquine Hydroxyurea Hydroxy- progesterone Hydroxyzine	❖ Hydroxyl group usually ↑ water solubility → less likely to cross the blood-brain barrier ❖ Exception: Hydroxyzine still crosses due to overall lipophilic structure
iso-	Isomer = Molecule with the same chemical formula but a different arrangement of atoms in the molecule	Isosorbide Isotretinoin Isoflurane Isoniazid Isocarboxazid	❖ Greek isos = "equal" or "same", ❖ "ISO = Isomer or Identical core, Slight Offset" ❖ "ISO = Similar Structure, Opposite twist" ❖ "ISO = Same parts, different shape"
levo-	The version that rotates light to the left	Levofloxacin Levothyroxine Levodopa Levonorgestrel Levocetirizine Levomilnacipram	❖ LEVO- for left-handed ➤ opposite of DEX- ❖ Usually a cleaner version of an older drug that was a 50/50 mix ❖ Not necessarily a left-handed (S)-enantiomer – in some instances the (R)-enantiomer rotates light to the left
nitra- / nitro-	Contains a nitro functional group ($-NO_2$)	Nitroglycerin Nitrofurantoin Nitroprusside	❖ Often act via nitric oxide (NO) release → blood vessel dilation ❖ "Knight" or "Night" mnemonics
nor-	N-demethylated form (one fewer methyl group)	Nortriptyline Norepinephrine	❖ Often active metabolites with reduced potency or altered duration
phen-	Refers to a phenyl group (a 6-carbon benzene ring) which helps drugs cross blood-brain barrier	Phentermine Phenobarbital Phenytoin Phencyclidine	❖ "-phen" drugs affect the brain = central nervous system (CNS) ❖ "PHEN = "PHENomenal CNS effects"

pred-	Corticosteroid	Prednisone Prednisolone	❖ "Predator" mascots
sulfa-	Contain a sulfonamide group ($-SO_2NH_2$)	Sulfamethoxazole Sulfasalazine	❖ This is a specific sulfur-containing chemical structure, not just any sulfur
tretin-	Retinoid ➤ Form of Vitamin A	Tretinoin Isotretinoin	❖ t-RETINoid

Drug Suffixes Guide

Suffix	Drug Class	Example(s)	Background / Mnemonics
-afil	Phosphodiesterase 5 (PDE5) inhibitors ➤ Erection meds	Sildenafil Tadalafil Vardenafil	❖ "Fill a phallus" ❖ "Phil, the penis" ❖ "AFIL = Amplifies Flow In Libido"
-androlone	Anabolic steroid	Nandrolone Oxandrolone	❖ "ANDROLONE = androgen loan"
-apine	Atypical antipsychotics	Quetiapine Olanzapine Asenapine Clozapine	❖ "APINE = Atypical psychosis intervention" ❖ Atypical = not a typical D2 dopamine receptor-blocking antipsychotic ❖ From dibenzapine = two benzene rings
-azine	1st-gen antipsychotics / antiemetics	Chlorprom-azine Promethazine Perphenazine	❖ "AZINE = Anti-Zany" ❖ "AZINE = Antipsychotic zone" ❖ From phenothiazine ring structure
-barbital	Barbiturates ➤ sedatives	Phenobarbital Pentobarbital	❖ "Barbed wire" visual mnemonics ❖ From "barbituric acid"
-benazine	Vesicular monoamine transporter (VMAT) inhibitors ➤ Dopamine depleters for movement disorders	Tetrabenazine Deutetra-benazine Valbenazine	❖ "Bins" visual mnemonics (recycling bin mascots) ❖ "Benzene suppressing dopamine zings" ❖ From benzene ring + aromatic hydrazine

-caine	Local anesthetics	Lidocaine Bupivacaine Cocaine	❖ "CAINE = Cuts off pain" ❖ From Cocaine (from coca leaves), the first known local anesthetic
-capone	COMT inhibitors ➤ Parkinson's Disease	Entacapone Tolcapone	❖ "CAPONE stops COMT cops from busting dopamine"
-cillin	Penicillin antibiotics	Amoxicillin Penicillin Ampicillin Oxacillin	❖ "Killin' bacteria" ❖ "Ceiling" visual mnemonics ❖ Latin penicillus = brush = From brush-shaped mold under microscope
-conazole	Antifungals	Fluconazole Ketoconazole	❖ "CONAZOLE's goal: fungal control" ❖ From azole ring structure
-cycline	Tetracycline antibiotics	Doxycycline Minocycline Tetracycline	❖ "CYCLINE = cycling through ribosomes" ❖ "Cyclone" visual mnemonics ❖ From 4-ringed cyclic structure
-dazole	Antiparasitic / Antiprotozoal / Anthelmintic / Anaerobic antimicrobial	Metronidazole Albendazole Mebendazole Tinidazole	❖ "DAZOLE = Destroys Anaerobes, Zaps Organisms, Larvae, and Eggs" ❖ "Dazzle parasites with -dazoles" ❖ From azole ring structure
-dipine	Calcium channel blockers, dihydropyridine (DHP) type ➤ BP meds	Amlodipine Nifedipine Felodipine	❖ "Dipping blood pressure" ❖ "DHP = Dips High Pressure" ❖ From DIhydroPyridINE structure
-dopa	Dopaminergic drugs for Parkinson's Disease	Levodopa Carbidopa	❖ From dopamine ❖ "Don't park, son"(Parkinson's disease)
-dronate	Bisphosphonates ➤ bone-strengthening	Alendronate Risedronate	❖ "DRONATE = bones dominate" ❖ "DRONATE = drones down osteoclasts"
-fenac	Nonsteroidal anti-inflammatory drugs (NSAIDs, mostly eye drops)	Diclofenac Bromfenac Nepafenac	❖ "FENAC = Fights Eye iNflammation And Cornea" ❖ "FENAC = FEels Nice After Cornea burn"

-fenacin	Muscarinic antagonists ➤ anticholinergics for overactive bladder	Darifenacin Solifenacin	❖ "FENACIN = FENds off pee spasms" ❖ "Fenced-in" visual mnemonics
-floxacin	Fluoroquinolone antibiotics	Ciprofloxacin Levofloxacin	❖ "FLOX through DNA"
-giline	Monoamine Oxidase B (MAO-B) inhibitors	Selegiline Rasagiline	❖ "GILINE = Giving dopamine Life IN Extra-time"
-gliflozin	SGLT2 inhibitors ➤ diabetes meds	Dapagliflozin Empagliflozin	❖ "FLOZIN = Glucose flows in urine" ❖ "-in" for inhibitor
-gliptin	DPP-4 inhibitors ➤ diabetes meds	Sitagliptin Linagliptin Saxagliptin	❖ "The opposite of LIPTON sweet tea" → Teabag visual mnemonics ❖ "-GLiPtIN = GLP-1 intact"
-glitazone	TZDs ➤ diabetes meds	Pioglitazone Rosiglitazone	❖ "GLITAZONE = Glucose Into Tissues, Activating Zones" ❖ "Glitter zone" visual mnemonic
-idone	Atypical antipsychotics	Risperidone Ziprasidone Lurasidone Ziprasidone Iloperidone	❖ "Delusions? I'm DONE!" ❖ Atypical = not a typical D2 dopamine receptor-blocking antipsychotic
-ipramine	Tricyclic antidepressants (TCAs)	Imipramine Desipramine	❖ TCAs are the -triptylines and -ipramines
-lamide	Carbonic anhydrase inhibitors (CAIs) ➤ glaucoma meds	acetazolamide brinzolamide dorzolamide	❖ "LAMIDE = Lowers Alkali, Minimal Diuresis" – oral CAIs are mild diuretics that cause bicarbonate (HCO_3^-) loss in urine
-lutamide	Antiandrogens	Enzalutamide Bicalutamide	❖ "LUTAMIDE = Locks Up Testosterone, Tamed"
-mab*	Monoclonal antibodies	See -umab, -ximab, -zumab	❖ "MAB = Monoclonal AntiBody" ❖ "Maybe" in mnemonic phrases

-micin / -mycin	Macrolide or aminoglycoside antibiotics	Gentamicin Azithromycin Clarithromycin Erythromycin	❖ "-Mycin = Might kill microbes" ❖ "Mice in there" visual mnemonics
-mustine	Alkylating agents ➤ antineoplastic (cancer)	Carmustine Lomustine	❖ "MUSTard gas for cancer" ❖ "MUST kill DNA = alkylating damage"
-nib	Tyrosine kinase inhibitors ➤ cancer meds	Imatinib Osimertinib	❖ "NIB = Nibbles cell signals" ❖ "Nibbler" visual mnemonics
-nidine	Alpha-2 agonists ➤ BP meds ➤ muscle relaxants	Clonidine Tizanidine	❖ Derived from guanine, originally isolated from guano (bird/bat droppings) ❖ "-nidine = Nighttime BP down"
-olol	Beta blockers ➤ Blood pressure meds	Metoprolol Propranolol	❖ "LOLs lower pressure" ❖ Jester's hat visual mnemonics
-olone	Corticosteroids	Prednisolone Triamcinolone	❖ "-ONE = Owns inflammation"
-onide	Corticosteroids	Budesonide Fluocinonide	❖ "NIDE = Neutralizes Inflammatory Dermatitis & Edema"
-osin	Alpha-1 Blockers ➤ BP meds ➤ Benign prostatic hypertrophy (BPH) meds	Prazosin Tamsulosin Doxazosin Terazosin	❖ An invented suffix with no Latin root ❖ "-osin = Open Sphincter in BPH" (urinary sphincter, allowing urine flow) ❖ "Block α1, or sin"
-oxetine	SNRIs / SSRIs	Fluoxetine Duloxetine	❖ "XETINE = eXiting depression" ❖ "OXETINE = OXygenates mood"
-parin	Anticoagulants ➤ "blood thinners"	Heparin Enoxaparin	❖ "PARIN = Prevents ARterial INfarcts"
-phenir amine	Antihistamines	Pheniramine Brompheniramine	❖ "PHENIRAMINE = Phenyl + Amine" ❖ "Phenomenally Itchy? Relief Arrives" ❖ "Phriendly to runny nose"

-phylline	Methylxanthines ➤ bronchodilator	Theophylline Aminophylline	❖ "Feline" visual mnemonics
-piprazole	Partial D2 agonist antipsychotics	Aripiprazole Brexpiprazole	❖ "PIPRAZOLE = Partially Inhibits Psychosis Response"
-prazole	Proton pump inhibitors (stomach acid reducers)	Pantoprazole Omeprazole	❖ "Protons? ¡Olé! ...and they're gone"
-pril	Angiotensin Converting Enzyme (ACE) inhibitors ➤ blood pressure (BP) meds	Lisinopril Enalapril Benazepril Quinipril	❖ "April = ACE season" ❖ Easter-themed visual mnemonics ❖ Latin prilus = attached, because ACE inhibitors bind the enzyme
-profen	Nonsteroidal anti-inflammatory drugs (NSAIDs)	Ibuprofen Ketoprofen Flurbiprofen	❖ "Proficient pain meds" ❖ "PROFEN = PROstaglandin ENemy" ❖ From propionic acid ❖ "The N said..." visual mnemonics
-relin	Hypothalamic-releasing hormone (GnRH) agonists	Goserelin Sermorelin	❖ "RELIN = RELeasing hormone in LINe" ❖ "RELeasing LINe = endocrine stimulator"
-rubicin	Antineoplastic ➤ Cancer meds	Doxorubicin Idarubicin	❖ "BICIN = Biocidal" – kill cancer cells ❖ "Rude Bison" (buffalo) mascots
-sartan	Angiotensin II receptor blockers (ARBs) ➤ BP meds	Losartan Valsartan Olmesartan Telmisartan	❖ "SAR(t)AN" → Selective Angiotensin Receptor Antagonist ❖ The "satans" visual mnemonics
-semide	Loop diuretics ➤ "water pills"	Furosemide Torsemide	❖ "SEMIDE = See my pee!" ❖ "SEMIDE = Sodium Excretion with My Diuretic"
-sone	Steroids	Prednisone Fluticasone	❖ Steroids "own" inflammation!
-statin	Lipid-lowering agents	Atorvastatin Simvastatin Rosuvastatin	❖ "Statins flatten fat-in arteries" ❖ From Latin "statere" (to stop) ❖ "-in" for inhibitor

-stigmine	Acetylcholinesterase inhibitors	Neostigmine Rivastigmine	❖ "STIGMINE = Strengthens acetylcholine" ❖ "STIGMINE = Stops acetylcholine's grim end"
-terol	Beta-2 agonists ➤ bronchodilators	Albuterol Salmeterol	❖ "TEROL = Take air" ❖ "TEROL = Two lungs, air rolls in"
-tide	GLP-1 agonists ➤ diabetes meds	Semaglutide Liraglutide	❖ "GLUTIDE = glue tide / glucose tide"
-tidine	H2 antihistamines ➤ stomach acid reducers	Ranitidine Famotidine	❖ "To dine (without acid)"
-triptan	Migraine relievers	Sumatriptan Rizatriptan	❖ "Tripped on" visual mnemonics ❖ "Tript" from tryptamine-like structure
-triptyline	Tricyclic antidepressants (TCAs)	Amitriptyline Nortriptyline	❖ "TRIPtyline = Trippy antidepressant" ❖ From 3-ringed cyclic structure
-umab	Fully human monoclonal antibody	Adalimumab Dupilumab	❖ "u = you = human"
-vir	Antivirals	Acyclovir Oseltamivir	❖ From "virus"
-vudine	Nucleoside Reverse Transcriptase Inhibitors (NRTIs) ➤ HIV meds	Lamivudine Stavudine Telbivudine Zidovudine	❖ "VUDINE = Viral Unzipping INhibitor" → Unzipping is a metaphor for reading/copying the viral RNA into DNA ❖ TelBivudine is for hepatitis B, not for HIV
-xaban	Direct Factor Xa Inhibitors ➤ Direct Oral Anticoagulants (DOACs)	Apixaban Rivaroxaban Edoxaban	❖ "Bandana-wearing mascots = 'Xa is banned'"
-ximab	Chimeric monoclonal antibody	Rituximab Abciximab	❖ Chimeric (mouse/human hybrid) ❖ "xi = mixy"

-zepam	Benzodiazepines ➤ sedatives ➤ anxiety meds	Lorazepam Diazepam Clonazepam Temazepam	❖ "Benzo – never been so calm" ❖ PAM for Positive Allosteric Modulator (of GABA-A receptors) ❖ "PAM = Peace And Muscle-relaxation"
-zodone	Mixed-action antidepressants	Trazodone Nefazodone Vilazodone	❖ "ZODONE = Zzz + serotonin tone"
-zolam	Benzodiazepines ➤ sedatives ➤ anxiety meds	Alprazolam Midazolam Triazolam	❖ -zolam benzos are generally shorter-acting than -zepam benzos ❖ "ZOLAM = ZOnes Out LAst Minute stress"
-zumab	Humanized monoclonal antibody	Trastuzumab Lebrikizumab Ocrelizumab	❖ Mostly human, some mouse ❖ "zu = zoo = human in a zoo (still mostly human)"

*In 2021, the World Health Organization (WHO) revised monoclonal antibody naming conventions, retiring the traditional "-mab" suffix. It was replaced with more descriptive stems such as:

❖ "-tug" for unmodified immunoglobulins
❖ "-bart" for engineered/artificial antibodies
❖ "-mig" for multispecific antibodies
❖ "-ment" for antibody fragments lacking an Fc region

This change does not apply retroactively—existing "-mab" antibodies retain their original names.

Glossary

Latanoprost (XALATAN)	80	Paroxetine (PAXIL)	105	Tizanidine (ZANAFLEX)	107
Levothyroxine (SYNTHROID)	16	PAXIL (Paroxetine)	105	Topiramate (TOPAMAX)	97
LEXAPRO (Escitalopram)	28	PEPCID (Famotidine)	62	TOPROL XL (Metoprolol)	18
LIPITOR (Atorvastatin)	13	PERCOCET (Oxy/APAP)	111	Tramadol (ULTRAM)	68
Lisdexamfetamine (VYVANSE)	82	PLAVIX (Clopidogrel)	60	Trazodone (DESYREL)	31
Lisinopril (ZESTRIL)	15	Potassium chloride (K-TAB)	48	TRICOR (Fenofibrate)	101
Lisinopril + HCTZ	66	PRAVACHOL (Pravastatin)	50	TRULICITY (Dulaglutide)	87
LOPRESSOR (Metoprolol)	18	Pravastatin (PRAVACHOL)	50	TYLENOL (Acetaminophen)	115
LORATADINE (Claritin)	85	Prednisone	43	ULTRAM (Tramadol)	68
Lorazepam (ATIVAN)	94	Prefixes guide	116	Venlafaxine (EFFEXOR)	57
Losartan (COZAAR)	21	Pregabalin (LYRICA)	104	VENTOLIN HFA (Albuterol)	20
Losartan + HCTZ (HYZAAR)	88	PRILOSEC (Omeprazole)	22	VICODIN (Hydrocodone/APAP)	36
LYRICA (Pregabalin)	104	Propranolol (INDERAL)	90	VISTARIL (Hydroxyzine)	59
Meloxicam (MOBIC)	42	PROTONIX (Pantoprazole)	29	Vitamin B9 (Folic Acid)	78
Metformin (GLUCOPHAGE)	14	PROZAC (Fluoxetine)	35	Vitamin D2 (Ergocalciferol)	51
Methylphenidate (RITALIN)	45	QT prolongation	8	Vitamin D3 (Cholecalciferol)	75
Metoprolol (LOPRESSOR)	18	Quetiapine (SEROQUEL)	95	Vitamin K (Warfarin antidote)	98
MOBIC (Meloxicam)	42	Renal dosing	9	VOLTAREN (Diclofenac)	64
Montelukast (SINGULAIR)	30	RITALIN (Methylphenidate)	45	VYVANSE (Lisdexamfetamine)	82
MOTRIN (Ibuprofen)	46	Rivaroxaban (XARELTO)	103	Warfarin (COUMADIN)	98
Naproxen (ALEVE)	102	Rosuvastatin (CRESTOR)	26	WEGOVY (Semaglutide)	61
NEURONTIN (Gabapentin)	23	RYBELSUS (Semaglutide)	61	WELLBUTRIN (Bupropion)	34
NORCO (Hydrocodone/APAP)	36	Salmeterol + Fluticasone	72	XANAX (Alprazolam)	54
Norethindrone + EE	93	Semaglutide (OZEMPIC, etc)	61	XARELTO (Rivaroxaban)	103
Norgestimate + EE	112	SEROQUEL (Quetiapine)	95	Z-PAK (Azithromycin)	91
NORVASC (Amlodipine)	17	Serotonin syndrome	10	ZANAFLEX (Tizanidine)	107
NOVOLOG (Insulin Aspart)	89	Serotonin withdrawal	11	ZESTRIL (Lisinopril)	15
Off-label	8	Sertraline (ZOLOFT)	24	ZETIA (Ezetimibe)	92
Olmesartan (BENICAR)	110	Simvastatin (ZOCOR)	32	ZITHROMAX (Azithromycin)	91
Omeprazole (PRILOSEC)	22	SINGULAIR (Montelukast)	30	ZOCOR (Simvastatin)	32
Ondansetron (ZOFRAN)	74	Sitagliptin (JANUVIA)	99	ZOFRAN (Ondansetron)	74
Opioid withdrawal	8	Spironolactone (ALDACTONE)	65	ZOLOFT (Sertraline)	24
ORTHO TRI-CYCLEN	112	Suffixes guide	118	Zolpidem (AMBIEN)	79
Oxycodone	73	Sumatriptan (IMITREX)	108	ZYRTEC (Cetirizine)	56
Oxycodone/APAP	111	SYNTHROID (Levothyroxine)	16		
OZEMPIC (Semaglutide)	61	Tamsulosin (FLOMAX)	33